"In this groundbreaking book, Matthew Skinta, PhD, ABPP, approaches the use of Minority Stress Theory (MST), intersectionality, and process-based approaches to work with sexual and gender minorities (SGM). To this point, what is known about MST are the many ways it impacts the lives of SGM people. Skinta is the first to incorporate MST in clinical practice. This book is ideal for trainees and practicing mental health providers who are working with SGM clients. MST and intersectionality are theoretical approaches that have been used to understand the challenges faced by people with marginalized identities. Skinta eloquently describes how to apply process-based techniques to work with SGM clients. Rooted in sound theoretical design, Skinta has developed a work that will likely be considered a seminal work in years to come."

lore m. dickey, PhD, North Country HealthCare,
Bullhead City, Arizona

"This volume beautifully summarizes relevant research regarding minority stress and uses this to guide a functional contextual approach to treatment when working with SGM clients. The volume's introduction thoughtfully lays a foundation for its contents, highlighting specific themes and key concepts. It effectively illustrates the integration of science into clinical practice through a minority stress lens, utilizing case vignettes and concrete examples that will support and enhance the work of even seasoned mental health professionals. Therapeutic approaches notwithstanding, the concept of contextualism is embedded within its content, as it includes material related to evolving language, intragroup dynamics, intersectionality, and the landscape of SGM professionals, including ethical considerations when working with SGM communities. Unlike many other sources, these topics are not just mentioned, but thoughtfully explored and integrated throughout the entire book. This volume also explicitly and repeatedly communicates the important point regarding necessity of intervention both with SGM individuals in therapy and within the larger environment that negatively impacts them. As such, this volume will be exceptionally valuable to mental health professionals, as well as trainees."

Colleen A. Sloan, PhD, VA, Boston Healthcare System and
Assistant Professor of Psychiatry, Boston University
School of Medicine

"Dr. Matthew Skinta is the leading figure in ACT and contextual science, focused on work with sexual and gender minorities. This book is like having a private course with Dr. Skinta, as he shares his profound perspective and deep compassion with you, the reader. Among books in this area, I give Dr. Skinta's book my unreserved and highest recommendation."

Dennis Tirch, PhD, author of The *Compassionate-Mind Guide to Overcoming Anxiety*

"Until now, there have been limited resources for therapists seeking to understand and help their sexual and gender minority clients within a contextual behavioral framework. This book is packed full of useful information and case examples, undergirded by the most current science and theory in these important and rapidly evolving areas of psychological scholarship. As a clinical supervisor and diversity educator, I plan to make this required reading in my graduate courses."

Monnica T. Williams, PhD, ABPP, Canada Research Chair in Metal Health Disparities, University of Ottawa

"Contextual behavioral theories hold much promise to facilitate the integration of social identities, contextual experiences, and histories of people who are sexual and gender orientation minorities into clinical theory. However, in the psychological literature, the specific needs and experiences of SGM people have only recently been integrated into clinical contextual behavioral theory. This text does much to specifically outline how the social identities and social experiences of SGM people might be incorporated into these existing theoretical treatment models and key CBT constructs and practices. The intersectional approach used by this text is particularly beneficial to address the real-world complexity of experiences, social backgrounds, and salient identities that reflect the individuality of each client, and how the client's background and identities might influence their functioning. This texts builds upon existing models of minority stress, cultural humility, risk and resilience, and considerations of power and privilege for SGM people to describe how these multicultural frameworks might be utilized across a range of CBT therapies in an innovative, practical, supportive, and clinically useful way. The framework presented in this book will be helpful for seasoned practitioners as well as for students and beginning therapists who wish to build a culturally affirmative clinical practice that integrates empowering strategies when working with SGM clients."

Susan Torres-Harding, PhD, professor, Roosevelt University

"Matthew Skinta has provided all of us with a much-needed book. Packed with vignettes, practical examples, and descriptions of applied skills, the book is an incredibly useful tool for clinicians who already work with SGM clients and want to deepen their understanding of how identity-based oppression impacts on mental health. It is also a precious resource for students in clinical trainings who really want to learn how to conceptualize and alleviate the suffering derived from rejection, shame, interpersonal bias or discrimination. A timely book infused with human and clinical wisdom that greatly enhanced my understanding of what it means to be compassionate toward my vulnerability and intimate with myself and others, as a clinician and a human."

Nicola Petrocchi, PhD, Professor of Psychology, John Cabot University and founder of Compassionate Mind – ITALIA

"This book is an essential SGM psychology reference and a must read for any clinician or therapist in training! Dr. Skinta's expert approach in this well written and highly informed resource is on the cutting edge of evidence based SGM-affirming psychotherapies. This important book is a guide for those therapists and researchers who already have a basic foundation in SGM psychology and are looking to enhance and advance their work and provide treatment that is process based, individually focused, and centered on the most current research and effective therapeutic interventions."

Laura Silberstein-Tirch, PsyD, author of *How to Be Nice To Yourself*

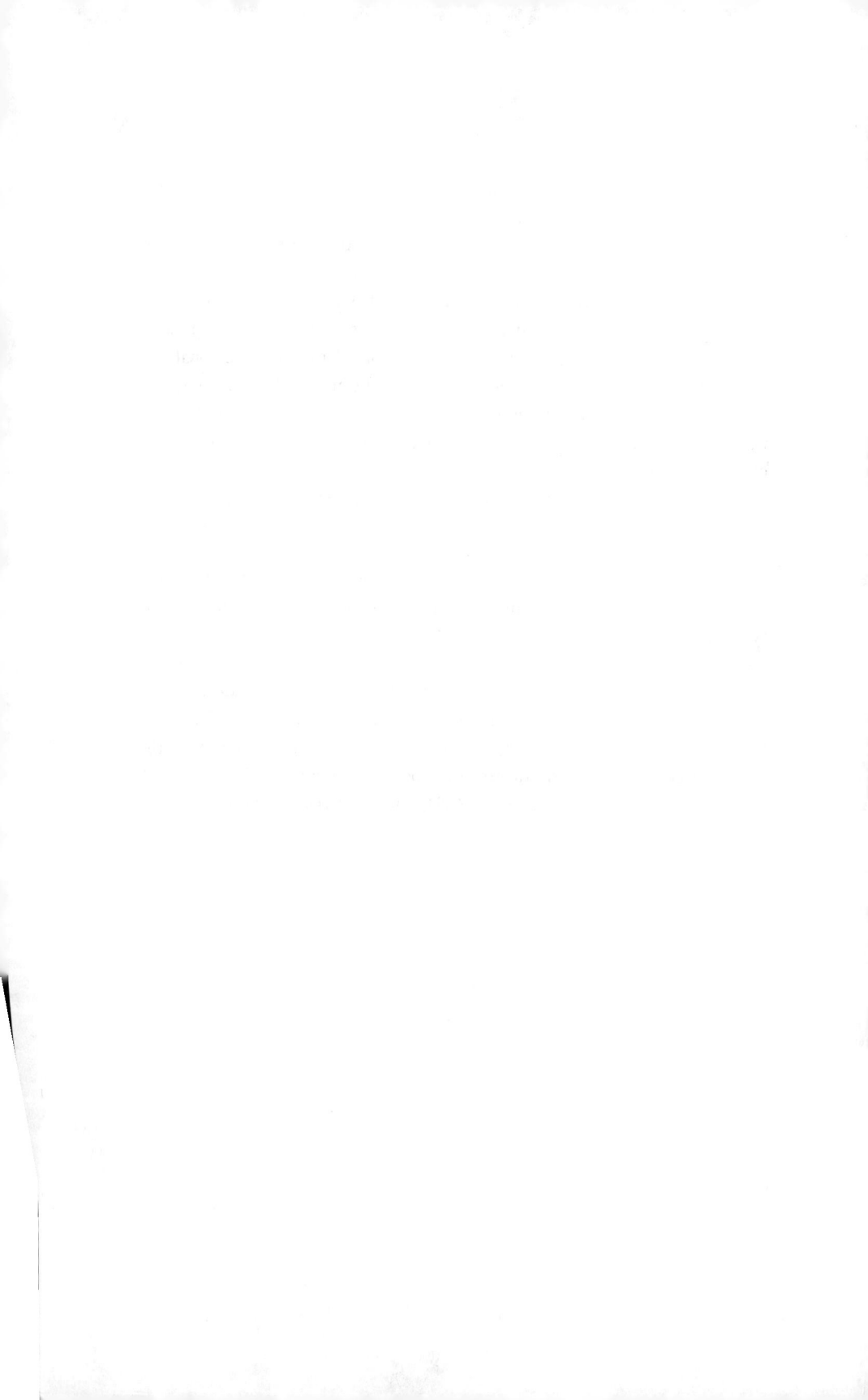

CONTEXTUAL BEHAVIOR THERAPY FOR SEXUAL AND GENDER MINORITY CLIENTS

Combining theory, research, and case studies, this book shows clinicians how to apply transdiagnostic contextual behavioral approaches when working with sexual and gender minority (SGM) clients.

The text first examines minority stress theory through the lens of contextual behavior analysis. Subsequent chapters illustrate the application of therapeutic techniques drawn from acceptance and commitment therapy, functional analytic psychotherapy, and compassion-focused therapy. The book concludes with a close look at special areas of consideration, including pre-surgical evaluation, the impact of HIV on SGM communities, ethical considerations, and future directions in therapy with SGM clients. Every chapter provides a series of diverse vignettes that illustrate how each aspect of treatment might build upon the last along with a list of recommended books for further exploration of that topic.

This book offers a unique, integrated approach that can be used for case conceptualization and followed as a treatment manual for professionals or graduate students with a foundation in SGM psychology.

Matthew D. Skinta, PhD, ABPP, is a board-certified clinical health psychologist and an assistant professor in the Department of Psychology at Roosevelt University.

CONTEXTUAL BEHAVIOR THERAPY FOR SEXUAL AND GENDER MINORITY CLIENTS

A Practical Guide to Treatment

Matthew D. Skinta

R Routledge
Taylor & Francis Group

NEW YORK AND LONDON

First published 2021
by Routledge
52 Vanderbilt Avenue, New York, NY 10017

and by Routledge
2 Park Square, Milton Park, Abingdon, Oxon, OX14 4RN

Routledge is an imprint of the Taylor & Francis Group, an Informa business

Library of Congress Cataloging-in-Publication Data
Names: Skinta, Matthew D., author.
Title: Contextual behavior therapy for gender and sexual minority
clients : a practical guide to treatment / Matthew D. Skinta.
Description: New York, NY : Routledge, 2021. | Includes
bibliographical references and index.
Identifiers: LCCN 2020026864 (print) | LCCN 2020026865
(ebook) | ISBN 9780367141196 (hardback) | ISBN
9780367141202 (paperback) | ISBN 9780429030307 (ebook)
Subjects: LCSH: Sexual minorities--Psychology. | Transgender
people--Psychology. | Context effects (Psychology) | Behaviorism
(Psychology)
Classification: LCC RC451.4.G39 S55 2021 (print) | LCC
RC451.4.G39 (ebook) | DDC 616.890086/6--dc23
LC record available at https://lccn.loc.gov/2020026864
LC ebook record available at https://lccn.loc.gov/2020026865

ISBN: 978-0-367-14119-6 (hbk)
ISBN: 978-0-367-14120-2 (pbk)
ISBN: 978-0-429-03030-7 (ebk)

Typeset in Joanna
by MPS Limited, Dehradun

To my husband, Barthélémy: Your enduring support helps make my work possible, and I cherish every moment of encouragement, distraction, and reminders for self-compassion. I am deeply indebted to every client, workshop attendee, consultee, supervisee, and supervised client that I have had the privilege of working with over the years. I am grateful to my supportive colleagues at Roosevelt University, who have given me the opportunity to stop wandering and begin to build. Every interaction has shaped how I convey these ideas, common barriers to implementation, and points of confusion. I have more mentors, role models, and supportive colleagues than I can name here.

CONTENTS

AUTHOR BIOGRAPHY

Matthew D. Skinta, PhD, ABPP, is a board-certified clinical health psychologist and an assistant professor in the Department of Psychology at Roosevelt University (Chicago, Illinois). He completed his PhD in clinical psychology at Kent State University, and a post-doctoral fellowship in HIV Behavioral Medicine at Harbor-UCLA Medical Center. He has conducted research at the UCSF Alliance Health Project, directed Palo Alto University's Sexual and Gender Identities Clinic, and maintained a private practice in the Castro neighborhood of San Francisco. Dr. Skinta has served on the American Psychological Association's ad hoc Committee on Psychology and AIDS, which he chaired for 2 years, and is currently completing a term on the APA Committee on Sexual Orientation and Gender Diversity. He is a peer-reviewed ACT trainer, a certified Functional Analytic Psychotherapy trainer, and a certified teacher of Compassion Cultivation Training. He conducts research on the interpersonal costs of minority stress upon sexual and gender minority (SGM) individuals as well as therapeutic approaches that promote vulnerability, acceptance, and self-compassion.

INTRODUCTION

This is an exciting time in the history of the psychology of sexual orientation and gender diversity. Decades of research on minority stress processes, the mechanism by which societal bias adversely impacts sexual and gender minority (SGM) people, offer great insights into the transdiagnostic processes that lead to psychological distress. The stage has been set to develop the next generation of SGM-affirming psychotherapies – interventions that incorporate the latest science in the service of supporting health and wellness regardless of diagnostic category that may benefit a wide variety of SGM individuals.

This book takes a *process-based* approach to the treatment of minority stress. That is, rather than a traditional cognitive behavior therapy manual that lays out a systematic approach to respond to a specific challenge or diagnosis, the goal here is to identify transdiagnostic targets and the corresponding therapeutic processes that a therapist might implement. The result is a flexible, customizable approach that may look different with each individual client, vary in the order of interventions selected, and highlight different aspects of therapy as they relate most specifically to the daily life challenges of the client.

Three broad concepts unify the content of this book: minority stress theory, intersectionality, and process-based psychotherapy. The first, minority stress theory, describes the array of stressors that result from anti-LGBTQ+ societal bias. Some of these stressors are internal responses to the world, like internalized stigma, while others are external, such as experiences of violence or discrimination. While current research suggests a great deal of overlap in the experience of minority stress across sexual orientation and gender identity, there are also some unique differences (Hendricks & Testa, 2012; Meyer, 1995). These are also not entirely distinct categories: not all sexual minority individuals are cisgender and not all gender minority individuals are heterosexual (e.g., Mizock & Hopwood, 2016). The second theme, intersectionality, emphasizes the importance of remembering that co-occurring minority identities are not divisible. For instance, a queer person of color who has experienced sexual racism (e.g., fetishism, stereotyping, or exclusion based on their race) is having an experience unique to both their sexual identity and their racial identity (Meyer & Ouellette, 2009). Many parts of the minority stress model may manifest differently for people of color, and these factors will be explored throughout. Finally, this book is framed around principles of process-based psychotherapy. Particularly for practitioners of cognitive behavior therapy, treatment manuals are presented as omnibus procedural guides and a manual is expected to be followed in a relatively standardized, linear format. In a process-based, contextual behavioral approach, the practitioner should feel free to explore and develop treatments only around experiences of the client.

The importance of language

Our use of language in professional contexts as we discuss sexual orientations and gender identities is incredibly important. The stage is set for a welcoming environment or microaggressions beginning with the intake paper work used in a practice or medical setting, through to the accuracy of language and pronouns in notes entered into the client's chart. Accurate language also changes over time, as both individuals and communities evolve in discovering language that feels more accurate. Mistakes will be made, and there is a possibility that some language used within this volume may become dated or no longer acceptable in the near future. Working with SGM communities, even for clinicians within the community, requires a blend of cultural humility and non-defensiveness, as well as a personal commitment to become familiar with all of your client's relevant identities.

In this book, you will find no walk-through or glossary of sexual orientations and gender identities. This is intentional. A few years back, while living in the San Francisco Bay Area near many of the world's current leading technology and software corporate giants, I learned of the trend of responding to questions that were particularly easy to find answers for with a link to the site "Let Me Google That For You" (www.lmgtfy.com). This site provides a link that depicts someone opening google.com, typing the question into the search window, followed by the results – a means of criticizing the very low amount of effort the questioner was willing to invest to find the answer. While I do think that novel or evolving terms for sexual orientations and gender identities may require discussions for mutual understanding, often the request for a quick reference is an expression of the belief that one can be relatively separate from, or unfamiliar with, SGM communities and still do this work well. While I certainly believe that a cisgender, heterosexual therapist can provide exceptional psychotherapy with an SGM client, I do not think this can occur without some effort on the therapist's part to understand the world their client inhabits. My general recommendation for those hoping to specialize clinically in working with SGM clients is to create time to stay current in both professional developments (either through research journals or relevant chapters of a professional organization), in addition to consuming pop culture media intended for SGM consumption. Further, a provider can always ask a client what a particular identity label means, though this may not provide enough information to interpret a client's behavior in the context of their life and community for the non-committed therapist.

This book presumes the reader has some basic familiarity with SGM communities, labels, and language, and feels confident in their ability to find information as needed. For that reader, this book can be a helpful tool for guiding clinical work, or a useful text for graduate students with a basic foundation in SGM psychology. Recommended books for further exploration will be provided at the end of each chapter for those wishing to explore a topic more deeply.

Chapter overview

The first part of this book creates a foundation for considering assessment and creating an optimal context for psychotherapy based on the existing literature. Chapter 1 explores how minority stress theory fits within a process-based approach to therapy, and how a functional analysis might drive treatment conceptualization. Chapter 2 considers the literature specific to the therapeutic relationship, as a necessary and powerful aspect of creating change. Considerations are explored regarding both the preferences and interpersonal needs of SGM clients and how they may differ from expectations related to heterosexual, cisgender clients, as well as the possibility of committing microaggressions against clients whose identities differ from your own.

Chapter 3 through Chapter 7 comprise the heart of the book, and break down components of therapy common across contextual behavioral approaches that correspond to transdiagnostic risk and resilience factors experienced by SGM clients: mindfulness and perspective-taking, acceptance and defusion, values and committed actions, vulnerability and intimacy, and compassion and community. Each chapter introduces a specific clinical skill, as well as illustrations of what this intervention might look like with a client. These chapters reconceptualize minority stress factors as specific points for clinical intervention, and a clinician reading this book might consider how different strategies can be combined in order to best meet the needs of individual clients.

The final section is organized around special topics, or areas that require additional attention in work with SGM clients: complex trauma and post-traumatic stress, health considerations, and ethical concerns. As research advances in the area of complex trauma, the unique histories of relationship ruptures and betrayal by key attachment figures maps closely onto the lived experiences of familial rejection so common among SGM individuals. Elements of treatment outlined in this manual bear some similarities to the sequenced, relationship-based approach advocated by some complex trauma researchers (Courtois & Ford, 2012). Other principles illustrated in earlier chapters have some demonstrated efficacy as a primary treatment for PTSD, or as a precursor to exposure-based therapies.

Health disparities affecting SGM clients have a number of drivers, and clinicians working in this area require some general competence and comfort in supporting and advocating for clients. SGM people report a variety of microaggressions or discriminatory acts in primary care settings, which worsen effective care and discourage contact with providers. Biobehavioral approaches that are unique or more common among SGM patients, such as PrEP adoption, HIV care, and gender affirming care are reviewed.

Regarding ethical practice in the area of SGM psychotherapy, much has been written though some areas of practice have not been updated in many years. How SGM communities organize themselves, differences in cultural practices around the possibility of multiple relationships, and the greater acceptance of SGM-identified providers being active members of their local community have all changed in recent years. Norms relative to personal disclosure in therapy by SGM therapists have also led to a variety of contradictory opinions. SGM individuals were early adopters of web-based and then phone-based dating platforms, for example, and these have quickly become one of the primary ways that some individuals find romantic partners or spouses (e.g., Rosenfeld & Thomas, 2012). Suggestions are made in this chapter regarding ethical practice and guidance on how such decisions might be approached.

The final chapter discusses future directions. While this book presents a clinical approach that is theoretically-grounded and draws on an extensive literature, it is also novel in many ways. There are no large, randomized clinical trials of the contextual behavioral approach presented here, and support for many of the component pieces are derived from a variety of experimental or small clinical pilot studies. There are also some areas of practice that are growing at a rapid rate, such as guidelines on work with gender creative children, that merit additional attention.

My hope is that this book might serve many purposes. While it could serve as a manual for a clinician to explore or challenge their current practice by, it may also serve as an inspiration to researchers who would like to strengthen support or build bridges through areas where the existing literature is unclear. It might also serve as a primary text for graduate students who are considering how they might conceptualize the therapies they are already learning, or who would like a template to consider what the robust minority stress literature means for their practice.

I would like to end with an acknowledgement of the debt this work owes to many mentors throughout my training. I've been inspired through the inspirational intersectional work and clinical skills of Mary Plummer

Louden and Khashayar Langroudi-Farhadi, consultation and experiences of deep vulnerability with Mavis Tsai, and Monnica T. Williams for her modeling of how best to respond to microaggressions as they occur within the routine practice of psychology and psychotherapy. My collaborator for many trainings across the globe and co-editor on a former book, Aisling Leonard-Curtin, remains a wonderful model and sounding board. My greatest thanks, however, extend to the dozens of supervisees and hundreds of workshop participants I have had over the years. They have challenged me to clarify and describe effective practice in ways that have led to this work, and through their own perspective and clinical work have broadened my understanding of what does and does not work.

Recommended reading

American Psychological Association. (2012). Guidelines for psychological practice with lesbian, gay, and bisexual clients. *The American Psychologist*, 67(1), 10–42.

Singh, A. E. & dickey, l. m. (2017). *Affirmative counseling and psychological practice with transgender and gender nonconforming clients*. American Psychological Association.

World Professional Association for Transgender Health. (2011). *Standards of care for the health of transsexual, transgender, and gender nonconforming people (7th ed.)*. Retrieved from https://www.wpath.org/media/cms/Documents/SOC%20v7/Standards%20of%20Care_V7%20Full%20Book_English.pdf.

References

Courtois, C. A., & Ford, J. D. (2012). *Treatment of complex trauma: A sequenced, relationship-based approach*. Guilford Press.

Hendricks, M. L., & Testa, R. J. (2012). A conceptual framework for clinical work with transgender and gender nonconforming clients: An adaptation of the Minority Stress Model. *Professional Psychology: Research and Practice*, 43(5), 460–467.

Meyer, I. H. (1995). Minority stress and mental health in gay men. *Journal of Health and Social Behavior*, 36(1), 38–56.

Meyer, I. H., & Ouellette, S. C. (2009). Unity and purpose at the intersections of racial/ethnic and sexual identities. In P. L. Hammack &

B. J. Cohler (Eds.), *The story of sexual identity: narrative perspectives on the gay and lesbian life course*. Oxford University Press.

Mizock, L., & Hopwood, R. (2016). Conflation and interdependence in the intersection of gender and sexuality among transgender individuals. *Psychology of Sexual Orientation and Gender Diversity, 3*(1), 93–103.

Rosenfeld, M. J., & Thomas, R. J. (2012). Searching for a mate: The rise of the Internet as a social intermediary. *American Sociological Review, 77*(4), 523–547.

1

A CONTEXTUAL BEHAVIORAL ANALYSIS OF MINORITY STRESS

Introduction

Minority stress theory has become one of the central lenses used to research psychological experiences of SGM populations (e.g., Graham et al., 2011). Minority stress theory began with the premise that anti-LGBTQ+ animus in society is ubiquitous and affects the well-being of SGM people in a variety of ways. No single measure, such as direct discrimination or internalized stigma (i.e., internalized homophobia, internalized biphobia, internalized transphobia), can capture the full impact of living in a biased society (Meyer, 1995). These factors are generally described as proximal to distal, and the list includes internalized stigma, rejection sensitivity, or the expectation of rejection, outness or concealment, discrimination or violence, and specific to gender minority individuals, being misgendered (e.g., referred to by an incorrect name or with incorrect pronouns; Hendricks & Testa, 2012; Meyer, 2003). More recent formulations include resilience factors, as well, such as community connectedness and, for gender minority individuals, pride (Hendricks & Testa, 2012; Meyer, 2015). Minority stress theory provides a starting point for case conceptualization and transdiagnostic assessment, and this chapter will explore how developing a minority stress informed treatment plan can be supported through a consideration of process-based therapy and a functional contextual approach.

The path to minority stress theory

In the first decades after the declassification of homosexuality from the DSM, most publications describing the sexual minority experience emphasized internalized stigma (i.e., internalized homophobia; e.g., Malyon, 1982). While a useful starting point as the field began to acknowledge the deleterious effects of pervasive anti-SGM bias in society, there were a number of shortcomings to this approach. First, the interpersonal and societal challenges facing SGM people were not contingent on resolving negative beliefs one was exposed to earlier in life. Familial rejection, social exclusion, and workplace discrimination all had harmful impacts, and it has been less than 20 years since the U.S. Supreme Court overturned the last sodomy laws that criminalized same-sex sexuality (for a broader discussion, see Eskridge, 2008).

This changed with the popularity of minority stress theory (Meyer, 1995). First described in *Minority Stress and Lesbian Women* in 1981 (Brooks, 1981), it was not widely adopted until subsequent promotion in the works of Ilan Meyer (1995; 2003). Based upon Brooks's grounding in systems theory, Brooks considered minority stress to be the biopsychosocial outcome of culturally sanctioned bias against SGM individuals, conveyed through both systemic bias as well as interpersonal interactions informed by anti-SGM animus (Rich et al., 2020). SGM individuals respond to the stress of living in a biased society in a number of ways, and minority stress theory offered enough flexibility to begin making sense of responses that ranged from anxiety to depression, substance use to sexual compulsivity (e.g., Lipson et al., 2019; Kerridge et al., 2017). Though initially minority stress research centered the experiences of and primarily included sexual minority individuals, the model was extended and refined to be inclusive of gender minority experiences (e.g., Testa et al., 2017).

The component parts of minority stress are internalized stigma, rejection sensitivity (or the expectation of stigma), concealment, discrimination, and violence, and in the case of gender minority stress, misgendering (Hendricks & Testa, 2012; Meyer, 2003). As noted in the introduction, it cannot be emphasized enough that minority stress is the response of SGM individuals to societal bias, and not a shortcoming of individuals (Meyer, 2019). In some cases, these may be adaptive responses to hostile environments. For example, concealment acts as a stressor, though may be an accurate response to a local context high in discrimination (Pachankis et al., 2015). Rejection sensitivity, which includes both interpersonal guardedness as well as a cognitive bias toward perceiving ambiguous responses as rejection or interpersonal submissiveness, may reduce unwanted attention in an environment in which safety is unclear (Pachankis et al., 2008). It must not be forgotten that targeting minority stress factors in psychotherapy is a means of healing individuals in societies that have not yet wholly embraced SGM people, and is not intended to supplant continued efforts to change society in ways that would allow SGM individuals to thrive (Meyer, 2019).

Research over the past decade has highlighted two major expansions of minority stress theory. First, most recent work incorporates a recognition of SGM-specific resilience factors into the model, as they mitigate the impact of bias in society (Meyer, 2015). Second, a series of studies has led to an emphasis on mediating psychological processes, with emotion dysregulation receiving the greatest attention (Hatzenbuehler, 2009). That is, the cumulative impact of minority stressors appears to diminish one's capacity for emotion regulation, which in turn increases the likelihood, varying by context, that an individual will experience adverse psychological and medical outcomes. This expanded model includes some elements not commonly listed though supported in the literature, such as experiential avoidance and shame as additional mediators, and self-compassion as a possible resilience factor (Figure 1.1; Gold et al., 2011; Leleux-Labarge et al., 2015; Mereish & Poteat, 2015; Vigna et al., 2018).

This model is incomplete, however. For SGM individuals with intersectional identities, one's lived experience is not simply minority stress plus racism, sexism, or xenophobia (Bowleg, 2008). While there have been fledgling attempts to measure intersectional stressors, such as the

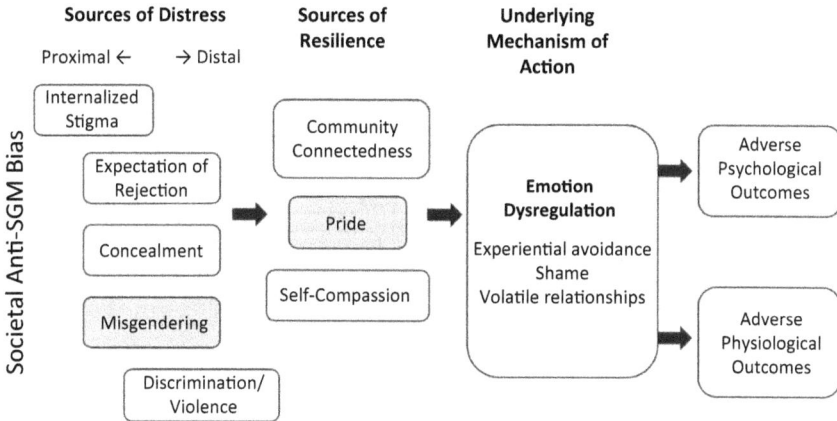

Figure 1.1 Minority stress model with proposed resilience factors and mechanism of action. Gender minority-specific factors are shaded.

presence of racism within SGM community spaces and anti-SGM bias with a community of color, it has been more challenging to identify ways to measure or assess responses to an individual as a whole person (e.g., Balsam et al., 2011). One example can be found in the growing literature on sexual racism, which appears to be an expression of covert racism (Callander et al., 2015). Sexual racism encapsulates those attitudes and expressions of attraction that either exclude or fetishize a person of color in SGM spaces, and serve as their own unique stressor (Han & Choi, 2018). Sexual racism among sexual minority men has been associated with higher body dissatisfaction (Bhambhani et al., 2019) and psychological distress (Bhambhani et al., 2020). For a consideration of factors missing from Figure 1.1, Figure 1.2 proposes some additional considerations for work with SGM people of color.

Finally, access to SGM communities may serve as stressors of their own. This can occur through pressure to identify with a particular label in the presence of identity confusion (Gandhi et al., 2016), anti-plurisexual sentiment, and bisexual erasure (e.g., Hertlein et al., 2016), and stress to conform to particular body standards (Frederick & Essayli, 2016). Finally, the term intraminority stress has been adopted to refer to those stressors that arise as a result of competition and status anxiety within communities of gay men (Pachankis et al., 2020). The minority stress model, as I hope these adaptations and addendum clarify, is still undergoing revisions

Sources of Distress

Proximal ←   → Distal

Sources of Resilience

Internalized Stigma re: unique race-based SGM stereotypes

Including connecting with SGM communities of color

Anticipation of racism within SGM community + *sexual racism*

Pride in one's whole identity

Meaning of concealment within meaningful POC communities

Additional microaggression or misgendering based on misogynoir

Higher rates of violence toward SGM POC

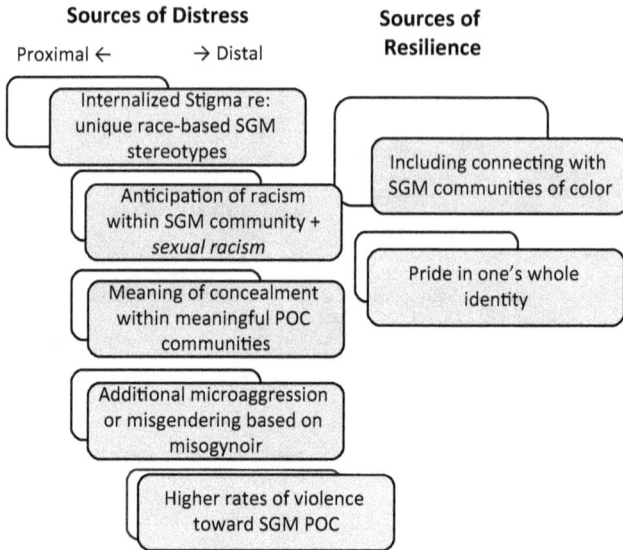

Figure 1.2 Emphasizing just the left side of the model, these proposed factors highlight intersectional interpretations of the minority stress model.

and refinements as additional work is completed. While the minority stress model serves as a helpful signpost in developing interventions, there is an array of individual factors that may arise in treatment that should be considered in determining the course of responding therapeutically.

Process-based therapy

In light of the recognition of common symptoms that do not correspond to specific diagnoses, and the recognition of transdiagnostic drivers of psychological diagnoses, many cognitive behavior therapists have shifted their attention toward process-based therapies (Hofmann & Hayes, 2019). Process-based CBT asks what core biopsychosocial processes presented by the client should be targeted, given their goals in their current context, and how might those be most efficiently and effectively changed (Hayes & Hofmann, 2018). In the case of minority stress, some early attempts have targeted emotion dysregulation as the underlying mechanism that may have the greatest impact, with some success in early trials with modifications of the Unified Protocol and Dialectical Behavior Therapy (e.g., Pachankis et al., 2015;

Sloan et al., 2017). While such a direction appears promising, there are additional ways to consider crafting interventions that are both mindful of minority stress theory as well as tools at the well-trained clinician's disposal. This has led to calls to develop and research interventions that emphasize SGM-specific treatment targets, such as internalized stigma, rejection sensitivity, and identity concealment (Cohen & Feinstein, 2020; Feinstein, 2019).

In exploring a contextual behavioral approach to treating minority stress, this volume sides with the latter argument. While a number of the skills and techniques that follow may be expected to also bolster emotion regulation skills, the emphasis is on dismantling some of the behaviors that developed as a function of internalized stigma, rejection sensitivity, and identity concealment. It is also worth recognizing that these are operationalizations that make these phenomena amenable to research, though they are not wholly discrete. For instance, cognitions about the world and other's responses to an SGM person found within internalized stigma may lead to some of the anticipated stigma that drives rejection sensitivity. Rejection sensitivity contains within the construct a number of behaviors intended to mitigate interpersonal rejection, that may be expressed through overly submissive behaviors, conflict avoidance, or interpersonal guardedness. Identity concealment, and the subsequent lack of interpersonal feedback that may undermine rejection sensitivity, are also deeply interconnected.

In this way, as the therapeutic interventions unfold in the following chapters, you may note that there are overlapping targets that are described. A mindful awareness of one's present environment may serve as a precursor to identity disclosure for some (Chapter 3), which may facilitate other vulnerable interpersonal disclosure that undermine rejection sensitivity (Chapter 6). Practicing self-compassion skills that soften the impact of situational shame may in turn lead to deeper relationships within the community (Chapter 7).

Developing a treatment that emphasizes transdiagnostic targets frees the evidence-based clinician from reliance on manualized therapies for contexts in which no clear manual exists without straying too far into the unknown. This is perhaps more important in working with SGM clients, as SGM individuals seek therapy at disproportionally high rates compared to the general population, and therapy seeking is not specifically tied to meeting criteria for a specific disorder (Cochran et al., 2003). Minority stress theory has proposed a number of specific targets that merit further attention during the course of treatment.

Philosophy of treatment

The general approach of this book is informed by the philosophy of functional contextualism. Functionalism is a simple metaphor for understanding behavior: it is defined by its impact or effectiveness, and assumes that the same behavior may serve a different function in different situations. For instance, I may come out to a family member or friend with a goal of building trust or allowing our relationship to become mutually closer. This is different than if I were to come out while lobbying with my member of Congress, where the function may be to enforce my words as a member of a community of voters. Contextualism takes a more radical stance regarding how we define the background in which a behavior occurs. There are internal contexts, such as one's sexual orientation and gender identity, memories about close relationships, or beliefs about how the world works, that all set the stage for how an individual behaves. There are also external contexts, such as how a diagnosis shapes a medical provider's interactions with me, political debates in my state or country about SGM rights, or encounters with violence and discrimination.

A functional contextual approach assumes that there is no such thing as a behavior without this inner and outer environment shaping the desired function, and that all of our behavior is functional. A client seeking a legally required provider letter to support a gender affirming treatment who places daily calls to their therapist about the state of the letter could be acting within a context of anxiety about the outcome, responding to a history of medical providers who lacked follow-through, or a pragmatic concern about pending changes to their health insurance that may limit coverage for the desired intervention. The same behavior is uninterpretable outside of that context.

The SORC model of case conceptualization

Each technique-focused chapter that follows incorporates the Stimulus-Organism-Response-Consequence (SORC) model for guiding a functional analysis of the client's behavior (Goldfried & Sprafkin, 1976). This provides a framework for considering both the function and context of a behavior, and draws attention to both inner and outer contexts that help to interpret, predict, or shape behaviors. This helps to fold in the range of minority stress targets, as well, so we might consider the broadest societal level of anti-SGM animus to the most internal fears, traumatic responses, or negative thoughts about the world. We will use this model to consider where to focus in each case, and as a general framework to steer our curiosity and consider where to explore further with clients.

Stimulus

The S in the model, Stimulus, refers to all of the possible antecedent factors in the past or present affecting an individual's life. This includes the place they live, their family of origin, and historical sources of trauma. My own experience as a supervisee and supervisor leads me to consider diagnoses and current medications as important pieces of a client's situation. These have social meaning when they appear on a provider's chart, both to the provider and to clients. One example is the diagnosis of *gender dysphoria* – one client may consider this a positive step toward receiving desired interventions, whereas another client may experience this diagnosis as an aversive sign of gatekeeping; their providers will have similar ranges of responses.

Organism

Though it sounds strange to many in this anachronistic usage, behavioral models often use this term to refer to the individual. This is the aspect of the model that captures the internal world of a client. What thoughts, emotions, or experiences comprise the current inner world of the client? Organism factors may include an individual's experience of attraction toward other or similar genders, an inner sense of gender or lack of gender, or dysphoria within their body. If you are familiar with an "A-B-C" model of behaviorism – antecedent-behavior-consequence – both S and O may be antecedents in this approach to case conceptualization.

Response

The Response refers to what a client is doing in response to the Situation and Organism factors. This can involve internal behaviors in response to their life situation, such as escaping into fantasy or ruminating, or could include behavioral responses such as not answering the phone, or evaluating the gender expression of one's outfit each morning before braving the world. The response can involve substance use to meditation, workable solutions to those that interfere with one's life goals. For many clients, this is a mix.

Consequence

This is where we consider how others in a client's environment are responding to them. This could include responses of family, colleagues, or systems that they are involved in. It can also be beneficial here to include the responses that the therapist has to client behaviors. Chapter 4 will explore in detail how to use your responses as a guide to better understanding the client as well as a place for intervention. Breaking cycles of unworkable behaviors that have been reinforced in the past is the primary goal of conceptualizing a case in this way.

Table 1.1 illustrates the types of questions or content that a therapist might assess in building a functional analysis of the client's experiences. This table will be revisited, with client-specific content, in the vignettes that appear in each therapeutic process chapter. While the names and clients are not specific to any one client, they reflect over a decade of private practice and many years of supervising SGM clients, and will illustrate common expressions of minority stress that clients may report within therapy.

You may begin to see how experiences flow from a client's history and inner experiences to behavioral responses, and what factors within the environment may be maintaining those patterns. Most therapeutic interventions target the client's responses to their own history and inner experiences. In some cases, such as through advocating for a more affirming setting in a medical office, situational factors may be directly acted upon (see Chapter 8). Changing the consequences of interpersonal behaviors most often arises within the therapeutic relationship, however. While we will explore the ingredients of an effective relationship in Chapter 2, Chapter 6 will describe specific principles to guide the therapist in order to reinforce under-rehearsed new interpersonal behaviors. This could range from providing a warm context for coming out to responding genuinely and authentically to disclosures of microaggressions or experiences of loss that the client has not previously had the context to voice. More than one intervention strategy may be appropriate for any given treatment target, so

Table 1.1 A Prospective SORC for Conceptualizing a Client's Minority Stress-Related Experiences

Stimuli	Organism	Response	Consequence
How did the family respond to the client coming out? What is the current socio-political climate? Has the client experienced discrimination or violence due to their identity?	What are the client's negative beliefs about their sexual orientation or gender identity, including what it means about them or what it means for their life? Does the client interpret unclear responses as signs of rejection? Does the client report shame, or feelings of something wrong with the self? Is the client affected by trauma memories?	Does the client actively work to conceal their gender identity or sexual orientation? Does the client avoid unknown environments or people? Does the client engage in behaviors to distract from unwanted internal experiences? Does the client disconnect from meaningful relationships (either out of fear of rejection, or painful associations)?	How do others respond to the client's responses? What do the client's responses elicit in you, as the therapist? How do systems, including healthcare, employers, or schools, respond to the client's responses? Are the client's responses workable for them, in terms of reaching their stated goals?

as you explore, consider that many of the approaches may be done in tandem, and none are mutually exclusive.

Summary

- Sexual and Gender Minority Stress is a model that elucidates how societal bias harms SGM people, and does not reflect any inherent shortcomings among SGM individuals.
- Sexual and Gender Minority Stress models offer a helpful guide in identifying SGM-specific, transdiagnostic targets for intervention.
- Process-based therapy suggests a framework for considering how to approach transdiagnostic, non-specific targets in therapy using existing tools in a flexible way.

- A functional contextual model can facilitate identifying treatment targets while remaining mindful of the societal context in which a client's behaviors are occurring.

Recommended reading

Hatzenbuehler, M. L. (2009). How does sexual minority stigma "get under the skin"? A psychological mediation framework. *Psychological Bulletin, 135,* 707–730.

Hayes, S. C., & Hofmann, S. G. (Eds.). (2018). *Process-based CBT: The science and core clinical competencies of cognitive behavioral therapy.* New Harbinger Publications.

Hendricks, M. L., & Testa, R. J. (2012). A conceptual framework for clinical work with transgender and gender nonconforming clients: An adaptation of the Minority Stress Model. *Professional Psychology: Research and Practice, 43*(5), 460–467.

Meyer, I. H. (2003). Prejudice, social stress, and mental health in lesbian, gay, and bisexual populations: Conceptual issues and research evidence. *Psychological Bulletin, 129,* 674–697.

References

Balsam, K. F., Molina, Y., Beadnell, B., Simoni, J., & Walters, K. (2011). Measuring multiple minority stress: The LGBT People of Color Microaggressions Scale. *Cultural Diversity and Ethnic Minority Psychology, 17*(2), 163–174.

Bhambhani, Y., Flynn, M. K., Kellum, K. K., & Wilson, K. G. (2019). Examining sexual racism and body dissatisfaction among men of color who have sex with men: The moderating role of body image inflexibility. *Body Image, 28,* 142–148.

Bhambhani, Y., Flynn, M. K., Kellum, K. K., & Wilson, K. G. (2020). The role of psychological flexibility as a mediator between experienced sexual racism and psychological distress among men of color who have sex with men. *Archives of Sexual Behavior, 49*(2), 711–720.

Bowleg, L. (2008). When Black+ lesbian+ woman≠ Black lesbian woman: The methodological challenges of qualitative and quantitative intersectionality research. *Sex Roles, 59*(5–6), 312–325.

Brooks, V. R. (1981). *Minority Stress and Lesbian Women.* Lexington, MA: Lexington Press.

Callander, D., Newman, C. E., & Holt, M. (2015). Is sexual racism really racism? Distinguishing attitudes toward sexual racism and generic racism among gay and bisexual men. *Archives of Sexual Behavior, 44*(7), 1991–2000.

Cochran, S. D., Sullivan, J. G., & Mays, V. M. (2003). Prevalence of mental disorders, psychological distress, and mental health services use among lesbian, gay, and bisexual adults in the United States. *Journal of Consulting and Clinical Psychology, 71,* 53–61.

Cohen, J. M., & Feinstein, B. A. (2020). Adapting cognitive-behavioral strategies to meet the unique needs of sexual and gender minorities. *The Behavior Therapist, 43*(3), 81–86.

Eskridge, W. N. (2008). *Dishonorable passions: Sodomy laws in America, 1861–2003.* New York, NY: Penguin.

Feinstein, B. A. (2019). The rejection sensitivity model as a framework for understanding sexual minority mental health. *Archives of Sexual Behavior.* Advance online publication. Retrieved from https://doi.org/10.1007/s10508-019-1428-3.

Frederick, D. A., & Essayli, J. H. (2016). Male body image: The roles of sexual orientation and body mass index across five national U.S. Studies. *Psychology of Men & Masculinity, 17*(4), 336–351.

Gandhi, A., Luyckx, K., Goossens, L., Maitra, S., & Claes, L. (2016). Sociotropy, autonomy, and non-suicidal self-injury: The mediating role of identity confusion. *Personality and Individual Differences, 99,* 272–277.

Gold, S. D., Feinstein, B. A., Skidmore, W. C., & Marx, B. P. (2011). Childhood physical abuse, internalized homophobia, and experiential avoidance among lesbians and gay men. *Psychological Trauma: Theory, Research, Practice, and Policy, 3*(1), 50–60.

Goldfried, M. R., & Sprafkin, J. N. (1976). Behavioral personality assessment. In J. T. Spence, R. C. Carson & J. W. Thibaut (Eds.), *Behavioral approaches to therapy.* Morristown, NJ: General Learning Press.

Graham, R., Berkowitz, B., Blum, R., Bockting, W., Bradford, J., de Vries, B., & Makadon, H. (2011). *The health of lesbian, gay, bisexual, and transgender people: Building a foundation for better understanding.* Washington, DC: Institute of Medicine, 10, 13128.

Han, C. S., & Choi, K. H. (2018). Very few people say "No Whites": Gay men of color and the racial politics of desire. *Sociological Spectrum, 38*(3), 145–161.

Hatzenbuehler, M. L. (2009). How does sexual minority stigma "get under the skin"? A psychological mediation framework. *Psychological Bulletin, 135,* 707–730.

Hayes, S. C., & Hofmann, S. G. (Eds.). (2018). *Process-based CBT: The science and core clinical competencies of cognitive behavioral therapy.* Oakland, CA: New Harbinger Publications.

Hendricks, M. L., & Testa, R. J. (2012). A conceptual framework for clinical work with transgender and gender nonconforming clients: An adaptation of the Minority Stress Model. *Professional Psychology: Research and Practice, 43*(5), 460–467.

Hertlein, K. M., Hartwell, E. E., & Munns, M. E. (2016). Attitudes toward bisexuality according to sexual orientation and gender. *Journal of Bisexuality, 16*(3), 339–360.

Hofmann, S. G., & Hayes, S. C. (2019). The future of intervention science: Process-based therapy. *Clinical Psychological Science, 7*(1), 37–50.

Kerridge, B. T., Pickering, R. P., Saha, T. D., Ruan, W. J., Chou, S. P., Zhang, H., Jung, J., & Hasin, D. S. (2017). Prevalence, sociodemographic correlates and DSM-5 substance use disorders and other psychiatric disorders among sexual minorities in the United States. *Drug and Alcohol Dependence, 170*, 82–92.

Leleux-Labarge, K., Hatton, A. T., Goodnight, B. L., & Massuda, A. (2015). Psychological distress in sexual minorities: Examining the roles of self-concealment and psychological inflexibility. *Journal of Gay & Lesbian Mental Health, 19*(1), 40–54.

Lipson, S. K., Raifman, J., Abelson, S., & Reisner, S. L. (2019). Gender minority mental health in the US: Results of a national survey on college campuses. *American Journal of Preventive Medicine, 57*(3), 293–301.

Malyon, A. K. (1982). Psychotherapeutic implications of internalized homophobia in gay men. *Journal of Homosexuality, 7*(2–3), 59–69.

Mereish, E. H., & Poteat, V. P. (2015). A relational model of sexual minority mental and physical health: The negative effects of shame on relationships, loneliness, and health. *Journal of Counseling Psychology, 62*(3), 425–437.

Meyer, I. H. (1995). Minority stress and mental health in gay men. *Journal of Health and Social Behavior, 36*(1), 38–56.

Meyer, I. H. (2003). Prejudice, social stress, and mental health in lesbian, gay, and bisexual populations: Conceptual issues and research evidence. *Psychological Bulletin, 129*, 674–697.

Meyer, I. H. (2015). Resilience in the study of minority stress and health of sexual and gender minorities. *Psychology of Sexual Orientation and Gender Diversity, 2*(3), 209–213.

Meyer, I. H. (2019). Rejection sensitivity and minority stress: A challenge for clinicians and interventionists. *Archives of Sexual Behavior*, 1–3. Advance online publication. Retrieved from https://doi.org/10.1007/s10508-019-1428-3.

Pachankis, J. E., Clark, K. A., Burton, C. L., Hughto, J. M. W., Bränström, R., & Keene, D. E. (2020). Sex, status, competition, and exclusion: Intraminority stress from within the gay community and gay and bisexual men's mental health. *Journal of Personality and Social Psychology*. Advance online publication. Retrieved from https://doi.org/10.1037/pspp0000282.

Pachankis, J. E., Goldfried, M. R., & Ramrattan, M. E. (2008). Extension of the rejection sensitivity construct to the interpersonal functioning of gay men. *Journal of Consulting and Clinical Psychology*, 76(2), 306–317.

Pachankis, J. E., Hatzenbuehler, M. L., Hickson, F., Weatherburn, P., Berg, R. C., Marcus, U., & Schmidt, A. J. (2015). Hidden from health: structural stigma, sexual orientation concealment, and HIV across 38 countries in the European MSM Internet Survey. *AIDS*, 29(10), 1239.

Pachankis, J. E., Hatzenbuehler, M. L., Rendina, H. J., Safren, S. A., & Parsons, J. T. (2015). LGB-affirmative cognitive-behavioral therapy for young adult gay and bisexual men: A randomized controlled trial of a transdiagnostic minority stress approach. *Journal of Consulting and Clinical Psychology*, 83(5), 875–889.

Rich, A. J., Salway, T., Scheim, A., & Poteat, T. (2020). Sexual Minority Stress Theory: Remembering and honoring the work of Virginia Brooks. *LGBT Health*, 7(3), 124–127.

Sloan, C. A., Berke, D. S., & Shipherd, J. C. (2017). Utilizing a dialectical framework to inform conceptualization and treatment of clinical distress in transgender individuals. *Professional Psychology: Research and Practice*, 48(5), 301–309.

Testa, R. J., Michaels, M. S., Bliss, W., Rogers, M. L., Balsam, K. F., & Joiner, T. (2017). Suicidal ideation in transgender people: Gender minority stress and interpersonal theory factors. *Journal of Abnormal Psychology*, 126(1), 125–136.

Vigna, A. J., Poehlmann-Tynan, J., & Koenig, B. W. (2018). Does self-compassion facilitate resilience to stigma? A school-based study of sexual and gender minority youth. *Mindfulness*, 9(3), 914–924.

2

THE THERAPEUTIC RELATIONSHIP AND CLINICIAN SELF-WORK

Introduction

Before introducing specific processes, the role of the therapeutic relationship merits particular attention. Separate from any particular theory or therapeutic modality, much of the early research on SGM psychotherapy emphasized the importance of an affirmative stance that would not lead to a reenactment of bias that SGM clients already experienced in their daily lives (e.g., Bieschke et al., 2007). Affirmative psychotherapy has been expanded in a variety of ways, however, and has been used to describe being knowledgeable about the correct language and history of SGM communities, a stance that normalized SGM experiences in non-pathologizing ways, and as an awareness of and avoidance of common slights (e.g., Burkell & Goldfried, 2006; Johnson, 2012). On a deeper level, however, the therapeutic relationship between a therapist and client, particularly when that therapist identifies as heterosexual and cisgender, recognizes the inherent power imbalance between a client and their therapist and the unique role that the pathologization of SGM identities play in broader, cultural forms of anti-SGM bias. This may be expressed through the identification of targets in psychotherapy and the relative weight given to the role one's sexual orientation and gender identity when presenting for care. An SGM client may also experience the opposite phenomena – as one older study notes, it is not uncommon that a sexual minority client might feel that their heterosexual therapist is affirming, albeit clueless as to how sexual orientation should fit into therapy (Mair & Izzard, 2001).

Ultimately, the past emphasis on affirmative psychotherapy has always described an atheoretical therapeutic approach rather than a psychotherapy, with past critics noting that for the field to grow, greater attention must be paid to the processes and outcomes of therapy with SGM individuals (Perez, 2007). While the emphasis of this book may suggest a bias toward always considering the role of minority stress, how this is explored within a particular therapeutic relationship can create either rupture or closeness. SGM clients also attend therapy at a higher rate than the general population, so the possibility that a client will come to therapy having past experiences of shame, microaggressions, or boundary violations from a therapist may be more likely (e.g., Mair, 2003).

There are also challenges of a different sort for those providers who identify as members of an SGM community. The perception of the therapist as reserved or transparent, vulnerable or closed, may mirror challenges a client has faced in their own history. A white therapist born within the United States who speaks English as a first language may fail to grasp the nuances of outness or feelings of belonging within the local SGM community by a client of color, or one who has migrated to the United States. There is also a possibility that a therapeutic stance of avoiding personal disclosures may inadvertently be perceived as modeling shame or discomfort when the therapist and client share an identity. There are also generational differences in community attitudes related to relationship norms (e.g., Hunt et al., 2019), HIV risks and the experience of living with HIV (Hammack et al., 2019), and the experience of internalized transphobia (e.g., Jackman et al., 2018). When unexamined, these differences may pose unique challenges to the therapy that would not be present among a dyad that does not share an identity.

This is not to suggest that the broader body of cognitive behavioral therapies do not benefit from a specific attention to the therapeutic relationship. In more manualized approaches, the critique has frequently been levied that an overreliance or emphasis on the specific tools of the approach may detract from the collaborative and supportive nature intrinsic in any therapeutic endeavor (e.g., Leahy, 2008). More recent guides have emphasized ways that the clinician may be mindful of the role of the relationship inherent in specific CBT competencies (e.g., Kazantzis et al., 2017). There is also support for the intentional addition of techniques that emphasize the role of the therapeutic relationship within a manualized approach (e.g., Kohlenberg et al., 2002). Though the emphasis in this book is on the use of process-based interventions, this does not ensure that a clinician will avoid an overreliance on techniques and activities over their experience with the client in a particular moment. This chapter provides a deeper exploration of the therapeutic relationship as the context behavior change might occur in, separate from any specific approach to therapy.

Working alliance versus the real relationship

One of the more popular constructs used to study the therapeutic relationship is the concept of a working alliance. As measured by the Working Alliance Inventory (WAI), it consists of three subscales: agreement on goals, alignment on therapeutic tasks, and bond (Hatcher & Gillaspy, 2006), and reflects the degree of collaborative agreement necessary for therapy to proceed successfully. Research specific to SGM clients supports the role of the therapeutic relationship as a mediator between affirmative practice and psychological well-being (Alessi et al., 2019). This study is of note as it also used the Real Relationship Inventory-Client Form (RRI-C; Kelley et al., 2010). The real relationship, in contrast with the working alliance, is a measure of the degree of perceived genuineness between two individuals, and the sense that they mutually view one another in a positive light (Gelso, 2011). Though the real relationship is generally correlated with the bond subscale of the WAI, this particular study specific to SGM clients noted that the correlations between the WAI and RRI-C across all subscales exceeded 0.70, suggesting a single underlying relationship between therapist and client (Alessi et al., 2019).

One possible interpretation, albeit from limited data, is that personal genuineness has a greater impact on SGM clients. When considered against the common history of many SGM individuals of familial rejection or common interpersonal struggles associated with coming out, it is reasonable that SGM clients may respond to a genuinely warm and affirming relationship more strongly, and have a lower threshold for perceiving collaborative possibilities beyond a genuine bond. Some of this may relate to rejection sensitivity, and concomitant contingent self-worth. That is, a more interpersonally guarded therapist or a "blank slate" approach is particularly likely to be experienced as judgment or rejection. This information may be taken as a challenge to the individual provider to consider their willingness to behave in as authentic and genuine a manner as possible, sharing their authentic positive and negative responses with the client within an affirming context. Though specific techniques are discussed in Chapter 4, the start of an effective therapeutic relationship with SGM clients is the setting of an intention toward authentically connecting with the client. It should be noted that prior studies also suggest that while sexual minority clients often rate gay or lesbian therapists as more helpful, there are not systematic differences by sexual orientation in client-reported measures of the working alliance or real relationship (Kelley, 2015).

What do SGM clients want?

Some studies have also explored the preferences of SGM clients in seeking psychotherapy. Though this chapter emphasizes the importance of the therapeutic relationship, it may be similarly meaningful to consider the preferences of SGM people. One recent survey that provided explanatory material on a variety of traditional approaches found no difference between SGM and heterosexual, cisgender participants in a preference for CBT; this preference persisted when compared against a specifically sexual minority affirming approach (McCarrick et al., 2020). This speaks to the tension between the point above, of the salience of the relationship to SGM clients, a desire for an effective approach, and findings that SGM clients experience psychodynamic/psychoanalytic approaches as less helpful (Israel et al., 2008). SGM clients generally describe a preference for active therapies that blend a warm therapeutic relationship with specific skills, psychoeducation, and relevant therapist self-disclosure. A negative or harmful reaction to the client's SGM identity is described as equally unhelpful as assuming that a client has an SGM identity without asking or the client labeling their identity (Israel et al., 2008).

Microaggressions in the therapy room

In considering the relationship in therapy, it is important to note the risk of microaggressions arising during treatment. Microaggressions are the subtle insults that are characterized by their incidental nature, the ambiguous deniability of insulting or denigrating a targeted minority identity, and the psychological harm that they cause (Sue, 2010; Sue et al., 2007). Debates over the relative utility and scientific support for the concept of microaggressions have periodically arisen in the literature, though a helpful review of such critiques makes clear that such criticisms often center on the need to clarify the motives of perpetrators of microaggressions, when the observed harm to those with minority identities is well established and should be sufficient to merit attention (e.g., Williams, 2019; 2020). There is limited research into the experience of sexual orientation microaggressions in therapy, though common sexual orientation microaggressions are likely to occur (Nadal et al., 2010). One qualitative exploration noted a range of pathologizing experiences reported by sexual minority therapy clients, ranging from assumptions of pathology and stereotyping to warnings against the adoption of a sexual minority identity (Shelton & Delgado-Romero, 2011). While some clients report an overemphasis on the role of sexual orientation in psychotherapy, studies suggest an avoidance of the topic within session by heterosexual therapists is also problematic (Conley et al., 2001). Explorations of microaggressions in therapy with gender minority individuals have identified common experiences including a lack of respect for client identity, lack of competency, saliency of identity, and gatekeeping (Morris, 2020). Gatekeeping refers to the process by which a provider takes on the mantle of authority in determining a client's ability to proceed with gender-affirming medical interventions, and will be explored further in Chapter 8. There is also evidence that intersectional microaggressions increase the harm that an SGM individual of color will experience, such that each additional identity a client holds may become subject to microaggressions by a therapist unaware of their biases (e.g., Fattoracci et al., 2020).

In contrast to microaggressions, some scholars have begun to explore microaffirmations, or the incidental behaviors that support and reflect a valuing of a client's minority identity. A qualitative study of therapeutic microaffirmations with gender minority clients noted that beyond the absence of microaggressions, microaffirmations included the acknowledgment of cisnormativity, disruption of cisnormativity, and seeing authentic gender (Anzani et al., 2019).

Therapist self-work

There has been a more recent movement within the cognitive-behavioral therapy (CBT) literature to promote clinician self-work (Bennett-Levy et al., 2001), which is particularly emphasized in contextual behavioral approaches. Studies of therapist training and effectiveness in Acceptance and Commitment Therapy (ACT), for example, have found that the therapist's own capacity for mindfulness, acceptance, and less thought suppression were associated with effective learning and implementation of the model (Pakenham, 2015). Contextual behavioral therapists also utilize mindfulness, acceptance, and exposure techniques to a greater degree than traditional CBT therapists in therapy, which speaks to the common practice of therapists who use mindfulness techniques maintaining a personal mindfulness practice (Brown et al., 2011). In FAP, the model most associated with working within the therapeutic relationship (Chapter 6), the standard model of skill acquisition occurs in regularly offered 8-week training courses online. At the introductory level, these courses emphasize disclosure, particularly of painful life histories or loss, and practice opportunities for responding in warm, vulnerable ways. Changes among trainee behaviors have been found in both self-reported and observer-reported ratings (Kanter et al., 2013; Maitland et al., 2016), as well as increases in empathy (Keng et al., 2017). In examining the working alliance between clients receiving FAP or client-centered supportive therapy, FAP demonstrated a small to moderate increase, despite both approaches emphasizing alignment with the client (Maitland & Gaynor, 2016).

An additional form of self-practice and self-reflection necessary in this work is to self-educate about SGM communities. Even for an SGM therapist, it is important to be aware of your specific community's history and the unique experiences of SGM identities that you do not share. There is evidence that, regardless of years of experience or religiosity, affirmative therapy trainings that impart information about the lives of SGM people lead to increased knowledge and a reduction in bias (e.g., Pepping et al., 2018). Despite this, most therapists report a lack of training or SGM-specific knowledge (Dillon et al., 2004; Farmer et al., 2013).

In my experience directing a sexual and gender identities training clinic for 4 years, as well as experiences providing consultation, workshops, and courses to international audiences, I have become a proponent of self-practice and self-reflection for all therapists as they relate to their own experience of sexual orientation and gender identity. SGM providers have often considered their own identities and explored the impact of those identities in their life as all SGM people do, though may experience limited modeling or opportunities for exploration in their training. Likewise, while heterosexual, cisgender providers have received the same anti-SGM cultural training that leads to minority stress among SGM people, they have rarely interrogated the ways that heterocentrism and cissexism have been conveyed to them. Through considering the messages received as a child around how to engage with our gendered bodies, as well as how we are to relate sexually with those of other genders, all therapists would benefit. In my training program and in longer workshops, I introduce a model consistent with the supervision and training approach of FAP that has been incorporated into each training year (Callaghan, 2006; Tsai et al., 2009). FAP therapist training, for instance, often incorporates elements of personal disclosure in the context of group supervision. In this instance, rather than a common exercise labeled a "life history" that involves disclosing vulnerable highs and lows that have shaped your experiences and led to this moment in your life, supervisees were encouraged to reflect specifically on messages they have received related to their sexual orientation and gender identity. Most cisgender, heterosexual trainees are able to recall experiences of how they learned the roles expected of them with minimal prompting. While many prior trainees have immediately considered examples of how a same-gender parent expressed to them how to "be a man" or "be a woman," others struggle. Examples that have arisen through working closely with those who feel unaware of how they have learned to move through the world include feedback from a romantic partner about sexist attitudes, or reflecting on moments of hearing SGM-related slurs used as insults. Similarly, I encourage an exploration of films, books, and community organizations that emphasize SGM topics. It is difficult to conceive of a therapist reducing culturally ubiquitous heterocentrism and cissexism without the experience of recognizing that it has also shaped their own being, and that these processes are not an exclusive part of the human experience of SGM people. However the reader might consider self-growth in this area, I encourage the consideration of an open and curious stance toward one's own history.

Conclusion

Psychotherapy is widely utilized by SGM individuals, and many therapists will treat many SGM clients without any particular training or knowledge of SGM communities. This undermines the ability of the therapist to provide an affirming, genuine relationship with the client and increases the likelihood that the client will experience micro-aggressions during treatment. To the extent that this chapter approaches clinician factors separately from the techniques that may be used to work within the relationship (Chapter 6), it is incumbent upon clinicians who wish to practice in an ethical and informed manner to engage in self-practice and self-reflection. This may begin with an orientation toward practice guidelines from professional organizations, though clinicians may benefit from considering their own felt experience of learning rules about how to behave as a cisgender person or as a heterosexual.

Key points

- The therapeutic relationship enhances the impact of evidence-based approaches in psychotherapy, and may be particularly important to SGM clients.
- For SGM clients, there may be a preference toward cognitive behavioral therapies, including contextual behavior therapies, alongside a preference for a clinician who is affirming and appears genuinely committed to the therapy.
- Seeking training, as well as connecting more deeply with the therapeutic approach you practice, through self-practice and self-reflection, may increase the likelihood of interventions being presented in a manner that is both personal and relationally attuned.

Recommended reading

Chang, S. C., & Singh, A. A. (2018). *A clinician's guide to gender-affirming care: Working with transgender and gender nonconforming clients.* New Harbinger Publications.

Gilbert, P., & Leahy, R. L. (Eds.). (2007). *The therapeutic relationship in the cognitive behavioral psychotherapies.* Routledge.

Kolts, R. L., Bell, T., Bennett-Levy, J., & Irons, C. (2018). *Experiencing compassion-focused therapy from the inside out: A self-practice/self-reflection workbook for therapists.* Guilford Publications.

References

Alessi, E. J., Dillon, F. R., & Van Der Horn, R. (2019). The therapeutic relationship mediates the association between affirmative practice and psychological well-being among lesbian, gay, bisexual, and queer clients. *Psychotherapy, 56*(2), 229–240.

Anzani, A., Morris, E. R., & Galupo, M. P. (2019). From absence of microaggressions to seeing authentic gender: Transgender clients' experiences with microaffirmations in therapy. *Journal of LGBT Issues in Counseling, 13*(4), 258–275.

Bennett-Levy, J., Turner, F., Beaty, T., Smith, M., Paterson, B., & Farmer, S. (2001). The value of self-practice of cognitive therapy techniques and self-reflection in the training of cognitive therapists. *Behavioural and Cognitive Psychotherapy, 29*(2), 203–220.

Bieschke, K. J., Perez, R. M., & DeBord, K. A. (2007). *Handbook of counseling and psychotherapy with lesbian, gay, bisexual, and transgender clients.* American Psychological Association.

Brown, L. A., Gaudiano, B. A., & Miller, I. W. (2011). Investigating the similarities and differences between practitioners of second- and third-wave cognitive-behavioral therapies. *Behavior Modification, 35*(2), 187–200.

Burkell, L. A., & Goldfried, M. R. (2006). Therapist qualities preferred by sexual-minority individuals. *Psychotherapy: Theory, Research, Practice, Training, 43,* 32–49.

Callaghan, G. M. (2006). Functional analytic psychotherapy and supervision. *International Journal of Behavioral Consultation and Therapy, 2*(3), 416–431.

Chang, S. C., & Singh, A. A. (2018). *A clinician's guide to gender-affirming care: Working with transgender and gender nonconforming clients.* New Harbinger Publications.

Conley, T. D., Calhoun, C., Evett, S. R., & Devine, P. G. (2001). Mistakes that heterosexual people make when trying to appear non-prejudiced: The view from LGB people. *Journal of Homosexuality, 42*(2), 21–43.

Dillon, F. R., Worthington, R. L., Savoy, H. B., Rooney, S. C., Becker- Schutte, A., & Guerra, R. M. (2004). On becoming allies: A qualitative study of lesbian-, gay-, and bisexual-affirmative counselor training. *Counselor Education and Supervision, 43,* 162–178.

Farmer, L. B., Welfare, L. E., & Burge, P. L. (2013). Counselor competence with lesbian, gay, and bisexual clients: Differences among practice settings. *Journal of Multicultural Counseling and Development, 41,* 194–209.

Fattoracci, E. S. M., Revels-Macalinao, M., & Huynh, Q.-L. (2020). Greater than the sum of racism and heterosexism: Intersectional microaggressions toward racial/ethnic and sexual minority group members. *Cultural Diversity and Ethnic Minority Psychology.* Advance online publication. Retrieved from https://doi.org/10.1037/cdp0000329.

Gelso, C. J. (2011). *The real relationship in psychotherapy: The hidden foundation of change.* American Psychological Association.

Gilbert, P., & Leahy, R. L. (Eds.). (2007). *The therapeutic relationship in the cognitive behavioral psychotherapies.* Routledge.

Hammack, P. L., Toolis, E. E., Wilson, B. D. M., Clark, R. C., & Frost, D. M. (2019). Making meaning of the impact of pre-exposure prophylaxis (PrEP) on public health and sexual culture: Narratives of three generations of gay and bisexual men. *Archives of Sexual Behavior, 48,* 1041–1058.

Hatcher, R. L., & Gillaspy, J. A. (2006). Development and validation of a re-vised short version of the Working Alliance Inventory. *Psychotherapy Research, 16*(1), 12–25.

Hunt, G., Wang, L., Bacani, N., Card, K., Sereda, P., Lachowsky, N., Roth, E., Hogg, R., Moore, D., & Armstrong, H. (2019). Generational differences in sexual behaviour and partnering among gay, bisexual, and other men who have sex with men. *The Canadian Journal of Human Sexuality, 28*(2), 215–225.

Israel, T., Gorcheva, R., Walther, W. A., Sulzner, J. M., & Cohen, J. (2008). Therapists' helpful and unhelpful situations with LGBT clients: An ex-ploratory study. *Professional Psychology: Research and Practice, 39*(3), 361–368.

Jackman, K. B., Dolezal, C., & Bockting, W. O. (2018). Generational differences in internalized transnegativity and psychological distress among feminine spectrum transgender people. *LGBT health, 5*(1), 54–60.

Johnson, S. D. (2012). Gay affirmative psychotherapy with lesbian, gay, and bisexual individuals: Implications for contemporary psychotherapy research. *American Journal of Orthopsychiatry, 82*(4), 516–522.

Kanter, J. W., Tsai, M., Holman, G., & Koerner, K. (2013). Preliminary data from a randomized pilot study of web-based functional analytic psychotherapy therapist training. *Psychotherapy, 50*(2), 248–255.

Kazantzis, N., Dattilio, F. M., & Dobson, K. S. (2017). *The therapeutic relationship in cognitive-behavioral therapy: A clinician's guide.* Guilford Publications.

Kelley, F. A. (2015). The therapy relationship with lesbian and gay clients. *Psychotherapy, 52,* 113–118.

Kelley, F. A., Gelso, C. J., Fuertes, J. N., Marmarosh, C., & Lanier, S. H. (2010). The real relationship inventory: Development and psychometric investigation of the client form. *Psychotherapy: Theory, Research, Practice, Training, 47,* 540–553.

Keng, S. L., Waddington, E., Lin, X. B., Tan, M. S. Q., Henn-Haase, C., & Kanter, J. W. (2017). Effects of functional analytic psychotherapy therapist training on therapist factors among therapist trainees in Singapore: A randomized controlled trial. *Clinical Psychology & Psychotherapy, 24*(4), 1014–1027.

Kohlenberg, R. J., Kanter, J. W., Bolling, M. Y., Parker, C. R., & Tsai, M. (2002). Enhancing cognitive therapy for depression with functional analytic psychotherapy: Treatment guidelines and empirical findings. *Cognitive and Behavioral Practice, 9*(3), 213–229.

Kolts, R. L., Bell, T., Bennett-Levy, J., & Irons, C. (2018). *Experiencing compassion-focused therapy from the inside out: A self-practice/self-reflection workbook for therapists.* Guilford Publications.

Leahy, R. L. (2008). The therapeutic relationship in cognitive-behavioral therapy. *Behavioural and Cognitive Psychotherapy, 36*(6), 769–777.

Mair, D. (2003). Gay men's experiences of therapy. *Counselling and Psychotherapy Research, 3*(1), 33–41.

Mair, D., & Izzard, S. (2001). Grasping the nettle: Gay men's experiences in therapy. *Psychodynamic Counseling, 7,* 475–490.

Maitland, D. W. M., & Gaynor, S. T. (2016). Functional analytic psychotherapy compared with supportive listening: An alternating treatments design examining distinctiveness, session evaluations, and interpersonal functioning. *Behavior Analysis: Research and Practice, 16*(2), 52–64.

Maitland, D. W., Kanter, J. W., Tsai, M., Kuczynski, A. M., Manbeck, K. E., & Kohlenberg, R. J. (2016). Preliminary findings on the effects of online Functional Analytic Psychotherapy training on therapist competency. *The Psychological Record*, 66(4), 627–637.

McCarrick, S. M., Anderson, T., & McClintock, A. S. (2020). LGB individuals' preferences for psychotherapy theoretical orientations: Results from two studies. *Journal of Gay & Lesbian Social Services*, 32(3), 1–13.

Morris, E. R., Lindley, L. & Galupo, M. P. (2020). *"Better issues to focus on": Transgender microaggressions as ethical violations in therapy*. The Counseling Psychologist, 48(6), 883–915.

Nadal, K. L., Rivera, D. P., & Corpus, M. H. (2010). Sexual orientation and transgender microaggressions: Implications for mental health and counseling. In D. W. Sue (Ed.), *Microaggressions and marginality: Manifestation, dynamics, and impact* (pp. 217–240). John Wiley & Sons Inc.

Pakenham, K. I. (2015). Effects of acceptance and commitment therapy (ACT) training on clinical psychology trainee stress, therapist skills and attributes, and ACT processes. *Clinical Psychology & Psychotherapy*, 22(6), 647–655.

Pepping, C. A., Lyons, A., & Morris, E. M. (2018). Affirmative LGBT psychotherapy: Outcomes of a therapist training protocol. *Psychotherapy*, 55(1), 52–62.

Perez, R. M. (2007). The "boring"state of research and psychotherapy with lesbian, gay, bisexual, and transgender clients: Revisiting Barón. In K. Bieschke, R. Perez, & K. DeBord (Eds.), *Handbook of counseling and psychotherapy with lesbian, gay, bisexual and transgender clients* (pp. 399–418). American Psychological Association.

Shelton, K., & Delgado-Romero, E. A. (2011). Sexual orientation microaggressions: The experience of lesbian, gay, bisexual, and queer clients in psychotherapy. *Journal of Counseling Psychology*, 58(2), 210–221.

Sue, D. W. (2010). *Microaggressions in everyday life: Race, gender, and sexual orientation*. Hoboken, NJ: John Wiley & Sons.

Sue, D. W., Capodilupo, C. M., Torino, G. C., Bucceri, J. M., Holder, A., Nadal, K., & Esquilin, M. (2007). Racial microaggressions in everyday life: Implications for clinical practice. *American Psychologist*, 62(4), 271–286.

Tsai, M., Callaghan, G. M., Kohlenberg, R. J., Follette, W. C., & Darrow, S. M. (2009). Supervision and therapist self-development. In M. Tsai,

R. J. Kohlenberg, J. W. Kanter, B. Kohlenberg, W. C. Follette, & G. M. Callaghan (Eds.). *A guide to functional analytic psychotherapy: Awareness, courage, love, and behaviorism* (pp. 1–32). Springer Science + Business Media.

Williams, M. T. (2020). Microaggressions: Clarification, evidence, and impact. *Perspectives on Psychological Science, 15*(1), 3–26.

Williams, M. T. (2020). Psychology cannot afford to ignore the many harms caused by microaggressions. *Perspectives on Psychological Science, 15*(1), 38–43.

3

MINDFULNESS AND PERSPECTIVE TAKING

Introduction

Mindfulness, or the awareness of the present moment as a flow of thoughts, emotions, and sensations, is a central part of all contextual behavioral approaches, either formally or informally (Hayes & Hofmann, 2017). Jon Kabat-Zinn has said "Mindfulness means paying attention in a particular way: on purpose, in the present moment, and non-judgmentally" (Kabat-Zinn, 1994), which aligns with subsequent attempts to elaborate and formalize the construct within the field (e.g., Bishop et al., 2004). The program developed by Kabat-Zinn, Mindfulness-Based Stress Reduction (MBSR) is a systematic, formal training that has had the greatest influence on current models of teaching mindfulness, so merits particular attention (e.g., Kabat-Zinn, 2009). MBSR is presented as an 8-week, 2-hour course that introduced a formal practice of meditation on the breath, combined with gentle yoga, that was initially promoted as a means of improving functioning and decreasing reliance on medication for those living with chronic pain (Rosenzweig et al., 2010). Though an indirect path to applications to SGM work, the success of MBSR led to many large urban hospitals developing local MBSR programs that began to be made available to SGM populations as the HIV pandemic spread (Gayner et al., 2012). In fact, most SGM people who have experienced mindfulness interventions as a part of research have likely done so within the framework of stress reduction for those living with HIV (e.g., Riley & Kalichman, 2015). The success of MBSR's presentation of a secularized version of Buddhist meditation inspired the extension of these techniques to the treatment of borderline personality disorder as a module within dialectical behavior disorder (DBT; Linehan, 2018), depression relapse-prevention in Mindfulness-Based Cognitive Therapy (MBCT; Segal et al., 2002), and numerous others. Subsequent research has supported that a lengthy daily practice is not the only way that individuals can benefit from mindfulness, and for those who have no prior experience, relatively brief mindfulness exercises (less than 15 minutes) appear to also have positive effects (Hafenbrack et al., 2019). This chapter will explore the related processes of mindfulness and perspective-taking as a foundation for the intervention tools in subsequent chapters.

The role of rumination

The value of mindfulness is found, in part, in the beneficial reductions it leads to in rumination (Heeren & Philippot, 2011). Rumination involves the recurrence and attentional focus on thoughts and memories, predominantly those involving negative content or affect that may be painful to experience (Nolen-Hoeksema, 2000). As such, it has been found to underlie a heightened risk for depression and depressed affect, as well as a reduction in attentional flexibility to one's environment where the context may not present those feared outcomes to the extent that ruminated thought content predicts (e.g., Hong, 2007). In this chapter, mindfulness and perspective-taking will both be described in terms of ways that the individual can experience their sense of self, as well as the content of their thoughts, that are amenable to intervention and can reduce the harm that arises due to rumination and critical self-focus.

For SGM individuals, there are a number of specific ruminative subjects that may lead to greater vulnerability. The literature on sexual orientation rumination suggests that for those individuals concealing their sexual orientation or unclear of how they identify, sexual orientation rumination is a particular source of distress (Galupo & Bauerband, 2016). Such thoughts often involve feared outcomes of coming out or identifying as a sexual minority, which can become a source of anxious or depressive emotions for those at this stage of self-identity formation (Borders et al., 2014). Gender identity rumination has been found to mediate the relationship between gender congruence and appearance with self-worth (van den Brink, Vollmann, & van Weelie, 2019), and may also serve as an important area of clinical intervention. Neither sexual orientation nor gender identity rumination should be considered developmental processes that only affect those in the process of identity formation. Coming out, self-disclosure, or the responses to one's disclosures or gender appearance may serve as threatening antecedents at any point in an individual's life span. This risk may be heightened by limited access to gender-affirming medical services as well. Approximately 40% of gender minority individuals in the United States have limited access to such care, and when an individual is experiencing conflict with their gender congruence without the ability to take steps to increase that congruence, gender identity rumination is likely to increase or be maintained (Puckett et al., 2018).

As Chapter 7 will explore more fully, traumatic events also occur at a greater rate for SGM people than among the general population (e.g., Roberts et al., 2010). Intrusive thoughts and rumination regarding experiences of discrimination or violence pose similar threats to well-being (Pantalone et al., 2017). Though this is a growing area of research interest and not all avenues have been explored, it seems likely that rumination related to traumatic or discriminatory events may heighten the salience of sexual orientation or gender identity rumination in ways that also undermine self-worth (e.g., Galupo et al., 2020).

Ways of experiencing the self

Within relational frame theory (RFT), a behavioral approach to language that underlies and informs many contextual approaches, mindfulness and perspective-taking reflect two different ways that we might experience our sense of self in a given moment. Mindfulness, when considered a form of attending to the present moment, is defined within RFT as *self-as-process*. That is, through settling into the present moment, often initially through tasks such as following the breath, one is able to experience the self as a flow of thoughts, emotions, and physical sensations that is continuous and perpetually changing (McHugh et al., 2019). In some moments of breathing or positioning the body, the physical restrictions of a binder worn to flatten the breasts may be more or less apparent. Thoughts of rejection or hostile interactions may increase or lessen depending on whether one is engaged in a heated discussion about environmental policy versus a similarly heated debate over proposed "bathroom bills" (e.g., Platt & Milam, 2018) that may increase the future possibility of hostile confrontations in public restrooms for those whose gender identity or presentation is not immediately perceived as conforming to both societal norms and the sign on the door.

Perspective-taking has been described within an RFT framework as the *self-as-context*. It is possible to cultivate a deeper experiential awareness that the flow of thoughts, emotions, and sensations varies not only from moment to moment, but also from the perspective of an individual's past or future, from the perspective of an observer, or across contexts. In an RFT model of the self, perspective-taking is made possible through learning deictic frames – those perspectives that are not reducible to metaphor or external example, rather from the process of learning the verbal relationships between I and You, Here and There, or Now and Then. Practice exploring one's inner and outer experiences through these frames ("how would you 5 years ago in your home town view you today, here and now?") has been found to promote psychological flexibility, self-compassion, and reduced rumination (McHugh et al., 2019).

It can sound paradoxical at first, as both self-as-process and self-as-context may not seem immediately different from rumination. The alternate experience of the self within RFT is *self-as-content*, or the experience of the self as being formed by a set of beliefs or self-statements (Table 3.1). For example, those experiencing sexual orientation and gender identity rumination are already looking at themselves through the lens of a possible negative future outcome, rather than a flexible sense of those moments as holding the potential for unexpected, different experiences. Working directly with those thoughts will be explored further in Chapter 4 through a

Table 3.1 Experiences of the self

Self-as-Content	Self-as-Process	Self-as-Context
I am depressed.	My breathing is a bit shallow.	If my closeted 12-year-old self could see me now, he'd think I had the perfect life.
I am a gay man, so my colleagues don't respect me.	Thoughts about yesterday's fight I had with my boyfriend keep coming to mind, again and again.	
My relationships never work and I'll always be alone.	My chest feels a bit constricted, and I feel guarded.	
I will not be able to find work if I disclose my gender identity.		

discussion of defusion, though it can be important to consider that the negative content contained within sexual orientation and gender identity rumination generally involves an overreliance on scripted, stigmatizing messages that exist in popular culture.

Outcomes related to SGM mindfulness interventions

A number of studies have considered the application of mindfulness-based interventions for those living with HIV, with many participants identifying as gay or bisexual men, though the treatment targets have generally emphasized HIV-specific outcomes rather than minority stress targets (e.g., Riley & Kalichman, 2015). Specific interventions that target SGM people broadly are limited, however. One study of gender nonconforming individuals found that trait mindfulness moderated the relationship between self-identifying as gender nonconforming and psychological distress (Keng & Liew, 2017). Research on Women's Health and Mindfulness (WHAM) groups that recruited lesbian- and bisexual-identified women found positive changes in health behaviors (Ingraham et al., 2017). Pilot studies that target internalized stigma have incorporated mindfulness in Acceptance and Commitment Therapy (ACT) groups for sexual minorities (Yadavaia & Hayes, 2012) as well as a modified protocol to incorporate self-compassion meditation among mindfulness meditation in an ACT group for sexual minority men living with HIV (Skinta et al., 2015). Both yielded positive outcomes, though mindfulness was one among multiple interventions in both studies. Finally, there are some studies that have examined the buffering effect of mindfulness against depression in the presence of racial microaggressions (Shallcross & Spruill, 2018). These preliminary markers suggest that mindfulness may be an effective tool in mitigating the effects of bias.

Introducing mindfulness and perspective-taking in session

There are both formal and informal ways that a therapist might integrate these practices into session. A more formal approach, as is often described within DBT (Linehan, 2018) and compassion-focused therapy (CFT; Gilbert, 2010), would be to begin each session with a brief mindfulness meditation that orients the client to this present moment, including whatever physical sensations they are experiencing, and observation of passing thoughts or emotions that are currently vivid. Such meditations can easily incorporate perspective-taking practices, if desired, through visualization meditations that may include prompting a client to observe themselves as a child in a past memory and noting what thoughts, emotions, and sensations arise, or through encouraging a client to "try on" the thoughts and emotions experienced when viewing the self, in that moment, through the eyes of a past or future point in time. For clients who resonate with such formal practice, there are a number of publicly available recordings of meditations or smartphone apps that the client might be encouraged to use. I have also allowed clients to use their own recording device or cell phone to record guided meditations within session. This has the added advantage of reducing the possibility of heterocentric or ciscentric microaggressions experienced during such practices, as many commercial recordings use gendered language (he or she, not they) when prompting visualizations.

It should be noted that formal practice is not always an option or consistent with a client's preferences. In my clinical experience, some (though not all) clients who wear binders experience physical discomfort when attempting to breathe deeply or in following their breath. Similarly, drawing subtle attention to the body, as it shifts and slightly moves in response to breathing, may briefly heighten the experience of dysphoria. This may be related to specific factors within the moment, such as an awareness of masculine or feminine physical features that are experienced as dysphoric, or may be related to a history of trauma in which sinking into a fuller awareness of one's physical body is uncomfortable. In either case, it is incumbent upon a clinician introducing a formal practice to request consent prior to a mindfulness exercise, describe the process about to unfold, share and directly speak with the client about potential challenges, and to debrief after a formal mindfulness exercise to see what unexpected difficulties may have occurred.

Informal practices are just as valuable. These may include asking a client during a moment of rumination or during the report of an unpleasant event to share their feelings in that moment, with you in the office, or to observe what changes have occurred in their emotional state or physical body during the recollection of an unpleasant or stigmatizing experience. Through continued prompting and curiosity about the client's experience right now, in this moment, no explanation or rationale is needed – the felt sense that the impact of a memory changes over time and across contexts is directly experienced by the client in these moments. Informal practice can also be assigned while a client is outside of session out in the world. For instance, it may be helpful for a client who realizes how challenging it is for them to notice the present moment to set an alarm for a random time each day, as a prompt to take a few minutes to notice the sensation of their breath, to watch their thoughts flow by, and to notice what sensations or tensions are present in the body. Slowing down and observing one's experience in this way may also facilitate interoceptive awareness of one's body that can elicit clarity in one's gender identity (see Langer, 2019, for a broader discussion of this experience).

Perspective-taking and flexibility in noting how one experiences the self over time may be particularly meaningful for clients who don't experience their sexual orientation or gender identity as static and unchanging. There is no single standard or rule by which a person labels their identity based upon past or imagined sexual behaviors or gender expressions, and such flexibility over the lifespan is not wholly uncommon (Manley et al., 2015). In my clinical experience, it has not been uncommon for both plurisexual (e.g., bisexual, pansexual) and gender non-binary or genderfluid individuals to feel pressure from friends and loved ones to adopt and commit to a monosexual, binary gender label. This is not everyone's experience, however. Modeling a stance of openness and curiosity toward one's fluid experience of sexuality or gender can aid in creating an affirming environment for self-exploration.

The function of mindfulness and perspective-taking

When considered as a part of therapy for minority stress concerns, it is important to consider the function of introducing these practices into therapy. First, as noted above, it would have a positive impact on sexual orientation or gender identity rumination; this is a straightforward illustration of process-based therapy, as a transdiagnostic symptom (rumination) is being treated with a transdiagnostic therapeutic process (mindfulness). As described in terms of experiences of the self, mindfulness and perspective-taking also may undermine or loosen the impact of internalized stigmatizing thoughts that are a part of the experience of self-as-content.

Case example

Louisa is a 32-year-old cisgender Latinx queer woman who identifies as butch. She entered therapy following a recent breakup, and described challenges within her relationship with her mother ever since she came out to her almost a decade prior. Current life stressors involve an increase in microaggressions in the workplace. She works at a boutique in a trendy neighborhood, and as the gentrification has increased over the past few years, so have degrading comments. She feels both her brown skin and her short hair and confident, masculine presentation have made her a target for the more conservative, wealthy white customers new to the neighborhood. As evidence, she notes that after a perfect employment history of many years, her manager has received at least one customer complaint a week about Louisa for the past 3 months.

In session, the therapist might wish to begin sessions with a brief mindfulness exercise, calling the client's attention to the present moment, what emotions she is still carrying with her into the session, and what content is active in her mind. Often for clients who have little experience with mindfulness, this process of noticing what the mind is doing is a powerful experience – one can be both swept up in interactions and simultaneously replaying a stigmatizing insult in back of one's mind, affecting one's mood and ability to focus.

A variety of scripts and recordings are available through either manuals for mindfulness interventions cited above or online, though a basic introductory meditation at the start of a session may look like the following brief script:

Adopt a comfortable posture with both feet on the ground, an erect posture, and closed eyes or a soft gaze toward the ground if you prefer. Begin by following the breath – noting the coolness of the in-breath, and warmth of the out-breath, or noting a spot at the edge of the nostrils where you are best able to follow the sensation of in, and out ... not trying to do anything special with your thoughts or feelings, though as best you can, returning again and again to the sensation. Simply rest your awareness on the breath... Allow your awareness to spread to the rest of your body. Perhaps noticing how it shifts as you breathe. Scan slowly from head to toe, noticing any places of tension or tightness in how you are holding your body. You do not need to change anything, simply allow yourself to see what is already here – how you have carried yourself through the day. Now begin to see if you can notice the thoughts arising right now, like clouds in the sky or leaves floating past on a stream. See if you can connect with the part of yourself that can observe the thoughts as they pass, seeing if you can allow this to happen without becoming caught up in them. If you find yourself caught up in a thought, perhaps taking a moment to go back to the breath, and beginning again.

Such a script could stretch from 3 to 5 minutes, depending on your pacing and natural rhythm as you guide the client. In this case, consider this dialogue following an introductory mindfulness exercise with Louisa.

Therapist: What are you noticing now, as you've settled into this moment?

Louisa: I feel calmer. I hadn't been aware of how tense I was, and I kept thinking back to a moment with a customer at the shop yesterday. She had wanted my coworker, a more feminine blond woman, to help her look.

T: What is your mind telling you about this?

L: Just that she was judging me based on my appearance, and uncomfortable with me. It comes with all these other thoughts about why I moved to a bigger city with a large queer community, and how much things are changing. I wish

	I would have said something, but it was so overwhelming right then.
T:	How are these thoughts affecting you right now, in this moment?
L:	Well, it's a bit more settled. Like being here with you, in the office, feels very calm. I know I have plans to see some friends after. They're also queer Latinx women, so I know they'll support me and know what it's like to put up with this.
T:	What are you noticing in your body as you shift away from yesterday and are here with me now?
L:	I feel calmer. I noticed that some of the tension I had in my shoulders and my lower back relaxed.

Notice in this example that a number of processes are occurring. The body is being used as both a source of focus, through the breath or sensations within the body, as well as a site of exploration in considering the emotional impact that recent life has had on Louisa. Despite not being asked to change anything, only to settle into the moment, Louisa has found some respite in her awareness of how this present moment is different than the micro-aggression she experienced at work. Prompts such as distinguishing the "shift away from yesterday" incorporate an element of perspective-taking. Louisa yesterday in the store was experiencing some stress and guardedness in a difficult moment. Louisa today is experiencing calm, and aware of having surrounded herself in other moments, like today, among those who are supportive of her and her experiences. Though other interventions later in this book may build on this moment, the degree to which Louisa is prone to rumination can be undermined by formal practice in this way. The purpose here is not to minimize those moments, and further exploration could lead to additional proactive coping. The presence of rumination can block more active coping, if it continued as a primary response to discrimination in the moment. We can consider what this chain of behaviors looks like going back to the SORC introduced in Chapter 1 in Table 3.2.

With practice attending to the present moment, Louisa may notice more active ways to respond. While she asserted a wish to have said something, which is one option that could be rehearsed in session, she also may determine that this is not a supportive environment for her and explore

Table 3.2 SORC of the Function of Rumination

Stimulus	Organism	Response	Consequence
Louisa has experienced some distance from her mother since coming out, which may be echoed in other relationships in the family.	Louisa may be defining herself in stigmatizing ways as a queer woman of color, or recalling messages she has received about her ability to succeed.	Rumination on the microaggression she received at work.	Active coping, and attending to positive connections and opportunities in her life, may be foreclosed as a result of rumination.
Louisa's neighborhood is changing, and she increasingly experiences microaggressions associated with both her racial and sexual identities.	Louisa is experiencing recurrent thoughts about the behavior of a customer in the store. This experience may activate other memories of mistreatment she has experienced.		

alternatives, such as deciding which friends are most supportive to call after these types of interactions, or sharing her observation with a manager to see if there may be ways that she could be better supported in the workplace. The goal is not to foreclose options or predetermine the right one, the intervention at this point is to interfere with the cycle of microaggressions and subsequent rumination overwhelming her other abilities to cope and to thrive.

Key points

- Sexual orientation and gender identity rumination might be best approached through mindfulness and perspective-taking interventions.
- Mindfulness and perspective-taking interventions are associated with improved well-being and decreased rumination among SGM people.

- Mindfulness and perspective-taking are common elements that underlie many contextual behavioral approaches, and reflect a therapeutic stance that supports each of interventions described in the following chapters.

Recommended reading

Curtin, A., Diamond, L., & McHugh, L. (2016). Self and perspective taking for sexual minorities in a heteronormative world. In M. D. Skinta & A. Curtin (Eds.), *Mindfulness and acceptance for gender and sexual minorities: A clinician's guide to fostering compassion, connection, and equality using contextual strategies*. New Harbinger Publications.

McHugh, L., Stewart, I., & Almada, P. (2019). *A contextual behavioral guide to the self: Theory and practice*. New Harbinger Publications.

Langer, S. J. (2019). *Theorizing transgender identity for clinical practice*. Jessica Kingsley Publishers.

References

Bishop, S. R., Lau, M., Shapiro, S., Carlson, L., Anderson, N. D., Carmody, J., Segal, Z. V., Abbey, S., Speca, M., Velting, D. & Devins, G. (2004). Mindfulness: A proposed operational definition. *Clinical Psychology: Science and Practice, 11*(3), 230–241.

Borders, A., Guillén, L. A., & Meyer, I. H. (2014). Rumination, sexual orientation uncertainty, and psychological distress in sexual minority university students. *The Counseling Psychologist, 42*(4), 497–523.

Galupo, M. P., & Bauerband, L. A. (2016). Sexual orientation reflection and rumination scale: Development and psychometric evaluation. *Stigma and Health, 1*(1), 44–58.

Galupo, M. P., Pulice-Farrow, L., & Lindley, L. (2020). "Every time I get gendered male, I feel a pain in my chest": Understanding the social context for gender dysphoria. *Stigma and Health, 5*(2), 199–208.

Gayner, B., Esplen, M. J., DeRoche, P., Wong, J., Bishop, S., Kavanagh, L., & Butler, K. (2012). A randomized controlled trial of mindfulness-based stress reduction to manage affective symptoms and improve quality of life in gay men living with HIV. *Journal of Behavioral Medicine, 35*(3), 272–285.

Gilbert, P. (2010). *Compassion focused therapy: Distinctive features*. Routledge.

Hafenbrack, A. C., Cameron, L. D., Spreitzer, G. M., Zhang, C., Noval, L. J., &

Shaffakat, S. (2019). Helping people by being in the present: Mindfulness increases prosocial behavior. *Organizational Behavior and Human Decision Processes*. Advance article online. https://doi.org/10.1016/j.obhdp.2019.08.005.

Hayes, S. C., & Hofmann, S. G. (2017). The third wave of cognitive behavioral therapy and the rise of process-based care. *World Psychiatry*, *16*(3), 245.

Heeren, A., & Philippot, P. (2011). Changes in ruminative thinking mediate the clinical benefits of mindfulness: Preliminary findings. *Mindfulness*, *2*(1), 8–13.

Hong, R. Y. (2007). Worry and rumination: Differential associations with anxious and depressive symptoms and coping behavior. *Behaviour Research and Therapy*, *45*(2), 277–290.

wIngraham, N., Harbaktin, D., Lorvick, J., Plumb, M., & Minnis, A. M. (2017). Women's health and mindfulness (WHAM): A randomized intervention among older lesbian/bisexual women. *Health Promotion Practice*, *18*(3), 348–357.

Kabat-Zinn, J. (1994). *Wherever you go, there you are: Mindfulness meditation in everyday life*. Hachette Books.

Kabat-Zinn, J. (2009). *Full catastrophe living: Using the wisdom of your body and mind to face stress, pain, and illness*. Delta.

Keng, S. L., & Liew, K. W. L. (2017). Trait mindfulness and self-compassion as moderators of the association between gender nonconformity and psychological health. *Mindfulness*, *8*(3), 615–626.

Langer, S. J. (2019). *Theorizing transgender identity for clinical practice*. Jessica Kingsley Publishers.

Linehan, M. M. (2018). *Cognitive-behavioral treatment of borderline personality disorder* (2nd ed.) Guilford Publications.

Manley, M. H., Diamond, L. M., & van Anders, S. M. (2015). Polyamory, monoamory, and sexual fluidity: A longitudinal study of identity and sexual trajectories. *Psychology of Sexual Orientation and Gender Diversity*, *2*(2), 168–180.

McHugh, L., Stewart, I., & Almada, P. (2019). *A contextual behavioral guide to the self: Theory and practice*. New Harbinger Publications.

Nolen-Hoeksema, S. (2000). The role of rumination in depressive disorders and mixed anxiety/depressive symptoms. *Journal of Abnormal Psychology*, *109*(3), 504.

Pantalone, D. W., Valentine, S. E., & Shipherd, J. C. (2017). Working with survivors of trauma in the sexual minority and transgender and gender nonconforming populations. In K. A. DeBord, A. R. Fischer, K. J. Bieschke, & R. M. Perez (Eds.), *Handbook of sexual orientation and gender diversity in counseling and psychotherapy* (pp. 183–211). American Psychological Association.

Platt, L. F., & Milam, S. R. (2018). Public discomfort with gender appearance-inconsistent bathroom use: The oppressive bind of bathroom laws for transgender individuals. *Gender Issues*, 35(3), 181–201.

Puckett, J. A., Cleary, P., Rossman, K., Mustanski, B., & Newcomb, M. E. (2018). Barriers to gender-affirming care for transgender and gender non-conforming individuals. *Sexuality Research and Social Policy*, 15(1), 48–59.

Riley, K. E., & Kalichman, S. (2015). Mindfulness-based stress reduction for people living with HIV/AIDS: Preliminary review of intervention trial methodologies and findings. *Health Psychology Review*, 9(2), 224–243.

Roberts, A. L., Austin, S. B., Corliss, H. L., Vandermorris, A. K., & Koenen, K. C. (2010). Pervasive trauma exposure among US sexual orientation minority adults and risk of posttraumatic stress disorder. *American Journal of Public Health*, 100(12), 2433–2441.

Rosenzweig, S., Greeson, J. M., Reibel, D. K., Green, J. S., Jasser, S. A., & Beasley, D. (2010). Mindfulness-based stress reduction for chronic pain conditions: Variation in treatment outcomes and role of home meditation practice. *Journal of Psychosomatic Research*, 68(1), 29–36.

Segal, W., & Williams, J. M. G. Teasdale. (2002). *Mindfulness-based cognitive therapy for depression: A new approach to preventing relapse.* Guilford Press.

Shallcross, A. J., & Spruill, T. M. (2018). The protective role of mindfulness in the relationship between perceived discrimination and depression. *Mindfulness*, 9(4), 1100–1109.

Skinta, M. D., Lezama, M., Wells, G., & Dilley, J. W. (2015). Acceptance and compassion-based group therapy to reduce HIV stigma. *Cognitive and Behavioral Practice*, 22(4), 481–490.

van den Brink, F., Vollmann, M., & van Weelie, S. (2019). Relationships between transgender congruence, gender identity rumination, and self-esteem in transgender and gender-nonconforming individuals. *Psychology of Sexual Orientation and Gender Diversity*. Advance article online. http://dx.doi.org/10.1037/sgd0000357.

Yadavaia, J. E., & Hayes, S. C. (2012). Acceptance and commitment therapy for self-stigma around sexual orientation: A multiple baseline evaluation. *Cognitive and Behavioral Practice*, 19(4), 545–559.

4

ACCEPTANCE AND DEFUSION

Introduction

Acceptance is a core feature of many contextual behavioral approaches, though it can be challenging in its implications and use with clients. Acceptance refers to a stance of willingness to be with all of the thoughts, emotions, memories, and external aspects of one's current context that are accessible within the present moment, without attempting to push away or control the experience (Hayes et al., 2011). At its heart, acceptance is a radical stance, and creates fertile ground for both personal change and engaging in committed actions intended to change the world. The goal of acceptance is to combat experiential avoidance; this refers not only to avoidance or attempts to control exposure to unwanted thoughts, emotions, or behaviors, it is often accompanied by cognitive fusion to rules about how the world works that undermine or mask opportunities for choosing different ways to behave in the world (e.g., Dinis et al., 2015). Though there are certainly examples of cognitive disputation of internalized stigma cognitions yielding positive results (e.g., Austin et al., 2018), my personal preference is to respond to internalized stigma among SGM clients with acceptance and defusion. As described below, these approaches do not require those cognitions be engaged with or argued, and in a world where there are always ready sources of bad news, discrimination, or violence toward SGM people, disengaging from a need to directly combat those thoughts may be experienced as liberating.

Acceptance in practice

It is worth noting what acceptance is not. Acceptance as a therapeutic stance and intervention does not mean passivity toward the status quo, and is not intended as a hopeless stance toward one's experiences or context. There is precedence, for instance, for avoiding the word "acceptance" entirely when working with populations that find the word "acceptance" particularly evocative of messages to give up a desire for change. For instance, while ACT and contextual-cognitive behavior therapy (C-CBT) for pain are identical treatments, labeling this intervention C-CBT avoids conflict with clients who assume that they are being asked to accept that their life and subjective experience of pain will never change or that they should settle for the current quality of life that is experienced as unlivable (Feliu-Soler et al., 2018; Gilpin et al., 2019). Others have noted concerns with the use of the word "acceptance" when working with communities of color in the United States (e.g., Sloshower et al., 2020). In recent years, there has been near-constant coverage in the news cycle of Black individuals being murdered in the United States (Aymer, 2016), which could create added dissonance in the encouragement to accept. The purpose of these caveats is to remind the reader that there is a distinction between the process itself – allowing one's self to notice, without defense, what thoughts, emotions, and memories are arising in the present moment – and the word "acceptance," which may or may not be pragmatic to use.

Acceptance, like defusion described below, is difficult to parse out of contextual behavioral interventions such as ACT and DBT. In terms of the broader literature on psychological flexibility, there is support for interventions that utilize these approaches as treatments for a wide array of difficulties, including depression (Bai et al., 2020), anxiety (Twohig & Levin, 2017), substance use (Byrne et al., 2019), PTSD (Wharton et al., 2019), and personality disorders (Reyes-Ortega et al., 2019). Those studies that have examined the effectiveness of acceptance as a mechanism of action when delivered as a part of ACT within treatment do support its role (e.g., Lundgren et al., 2008).

Work that considers internalized stigma and experiential avoidance or acceptance among SGM individuals have supported its role as a mediator between psychological stressors and well-being, including the stress of sexual racism (e.g., Bhambhani et al., 2020, Puckett and Levitt, 2015). It is worth noting that the same measure, the Acceptance and Action Questions – II (AAQ-II; Bond et al., 2011) is referred to across studies as either psychological flexibility or experiential avoidance, depending on whether or not it is reverse-scored, and is the most commonly used measure to assess acceptance in ACT studies. Studies of ACT with SGM populations that have employed the AAQ-II have consistently demonstrated change toward psychological flexibility as a result of intervention, with concurrent reductions in internalized stigma, including HIV-related stigma (e.g., Skinta et al., 2015; Yadavaia & Hayes, 2012). Psychological flexiblity has also been associated with reduced work stress among sexual minority individuals (Singh & O'Brien, 2020).

Defusion in practice

Defusion refers to the process of uncoupling our human tendency to treat our thoughts as expressions of literal truth (fusion), with the goal of creating more freedom to both accept unwanted thoughts and to experience greater freedom in the behaviors our thoughts lead us toward (Blackledge, 2015). One example is to think of simple basic words, such as the word "chair." When I use the word "chair" to describe where I would like you to sit, or what I am asking you to carry or move, it is helpful to recognize that the word is associated with a specific object out in the world. The challenge with fusion arises in that our verbal worlds are both full of daily behaviors that reinforce treating words as having literal power, while also having thoughts or receiving messages such as "I will be pigeonholed and never able to advance in my career if I came out," that are not necessarily true, useful, or applicable across contexts.

Defusion may also be particularly meaningful for SGM individuals struggling to label their experiences or discover an identity that feels like a fit in their lives. With clients either exploring or experiencing difficulty inhabiting an identity, it is imperative to remember that defusion techniques are intended to deliteralize language, not contact with the external world. I was once consulted by a clinician new to ACT who had been engaging unsuccessfully in attempts to use defusion techniques with a gender minority client regarding physical features that they experienced as dysphoric. This would not be expected to work – contact with their own body would undermine such attempts – though the clinician may have been more successful exploring what thoughts these experiences of dysphoria gave rise to. For example, a non-binary AMAB (assigned male at birth) person with broad shoulders may experience distress related to their physical body, though defusion would target the thoughts this could give rise to, such as "I will not be accepted in enby (i.e., non-binary) spaces due to my broad shoulders," or "My body will prevent my family from using my correct pronouns." Experiencing these thoughts as literal aspects of the world, as completely believable, is the source of pain that may be targeted through defusion. A prompt that immediately raises awareness of the role of fusion for many clients is "What would be different about tomorrow if you woke up and found that thought particularly unbelievable, or not quite convincing? Would you feel or behave differently?"

Externalizing and accepting thoughts and feelings

One common practice in dissemination manuals for ACT is to take advantage of the tools of fusion and avoidance to undermine the literalness and avoidance of painful thoughts. This has been done through practices, for example asking a client to describe inner experiences, such as depression or anxiety, as if they were pulled from the body and could be held in whatever shape the client imagines, or in designating a household object as the painful thought to carry. For example, a client might carry a penny in their back pocket to represent persistent fear thoughts regarding someone discovering their sexual orientation. This practice of literally carrying the thought, and the experience of how their attention ebbs and flows between hyperawareness or forgetting the carried object, can allow a client contact with the lived experience that a painful thought may shift in its relative weight from moment to moment. Much like mindfully observing thoughts (Chapter 3), such experiences can help a client come in contact with the deeper realization that even painful thoughts vary in both believability and in the effect that they have on behavior. This is an important realization, as it creates space to consider that the problem is not the thought that persists, it is how the client behaves in the presence of that thought.

Thoughts on paper

There are a number of ways that one might encourage a client to explore externalizing persistent and painful thoughts in order to manipulate them outside of the echo chamber of the mind. I am deeply indebted to the creativity of past clients in exploring and developing techniques that I have had the opportunity to use with other clients. One of the most basic interventions that some clients have found helpful, particularly when distressed by a particular recurring thought, is to write it down on an index card or small piece of paper that they can either carry with them or post in a place they will periodically pass in the course of daily life, such as the bathroom mirror or a kitchen cupboard. After writing this thought, the client is asked to note somewhere else on the card how believable the thought is experienced, in that moment, from 0% to 100%. After this, the client's assignment is to note on the same card, every time they pass (or if they are carrying it with them, at preselected intervals during the day), how believable it is in that moment. It is often a short period of time before the client realizes that the card is holding a range of scores across the full range of believability, noted in their own handwriting. Experientially, it begins to undermine the impact of a thought in a difficult, more believable moment when confronted by this evidence of their shifting relationship with the thought. If this particularly painful thought is neither always believable nor always affecting their mood or behavior, the client can begin to consider if they would choose to behave differently in the presence of that thought.

Sometimes the challenge is not a single thought, it is the cacophony of self-doubts or self-stigmatizing beliefs that a client finds difficulty defusing from or allowing them access to what needs accepted in the present moment. Many clients have built from the prior example to write each thought on sticky notes, which can then be added in a private place as they arise – inside a locked drawer at work, on the inside of a cupboard, or even on the wall of a spare room. The ability to step back and notice the array of conflicting thoughts in their varied positions can be a powerful reminder of the unreliability of the mind's negative bias, particularly for those whose thoughts are self-critical. One former supervisee, Vinisha Rana, began to modify this approach with clients who were struggling with rigid beliefs related to their relationships. Rather than draw attention to the struggle between conflicting views of another – I love my mother, and my mother has made harmful comments about my sexual orientation and her religious beliefs that have been painful – each of those thoughts, positive and negative, can be written on a piece of paper and spread out over a surface to for viewing. Letting go of the struggle of finding a rigid, accurate position, seeing a note about a particularly loving memory or comment laid out alongside a hurtful comment provides space to see a relationship in all of its contradictions. After laying out a number of thoughts in this way, the client would be invited to allow their eyes to wander and to note the felt experience of viewing these thoughts and simply allowing themselves to let them all be somewhat true. This is not unlike the comma-and exercise I describe in another volume, that encourages the client to allow contradictory experiences and thoughts to coexist (Skinta & D'Alton, 2016).

A note on affirming practice

I am aware that these techniques have been used and described in some case studies, particularly by those oriented primarily toward religious identities, to attempt to practice defusing from experiences of attraction to the same gender or from experiences of gender dysphoria. In adhering to professional standards for affirmative practice, I would recommend against this. From the level of clinical experience, I question whether such approaches would be successful, as physiological arousal or interoceptive awareness of gendered features of the body may undermine the longtime utility of this approach. It also violates common guidelines for practice with SGM clients (for psychologists, see American Psychological Association, 2012; 2015), as it dismisses the ways in which variance in attraction and experiences of gender occur across populations, cultures, and time (Stief, 2017).

Case example

Rebecca is a 49-year-old cisgender White lesbian who entered therapy related to depression, difficulties adjusting to a difficult work environment, and health difficulties. She has enjoyed her job in graphic design for a number of years and received numerous promotions, and had lived most of her life in Minneapolis, where she was born and raised and had a large network of friends and family prior to being transferred to a new regional office in a small Southern town that was significantly more conservative. She identified as a "soft butch," and while she was out to her friends she did not typically discuss her sexual orientation at work and only came out to her family 10 years prior. Following the move, her new manager began to routinely comment on her short hair and lack of makeup, often making jokes implying that he knew she was a lesbian. Though she initially brushed these comments off, over time the tone of the jokes became increasingly barbed. She was concerned about finding other work in her field if she left without a new position lined up, and her company declined her attempt to transfer back to her former office. Separated from her community and enduring frequent, daily homophobia, her mood began to darken and she began periodically skipping medication she was prescribed for hypertension. This was dangerous, as her hypertension was diagnosed after she collapsed at work a few years prior and was found to have experienced an aortic rupture. At the time of her intake, she admitted that her lapses in taking her medication as prescribed had co-occurred with passive suicidal ideation, often experienced as a fleeting desire to have the depressive mood and work experiences stop.

Rebecca initially used her sessions to vent about the difficulties she was experiencing at work, the futility of finding alternatives, and her sense of being stuck and sinking deeper into quicksand. She described herself as historically optimistic, so often feigns the carefree, optimistic presentation her friends are used to when she receives calls from her old friends from home or from family. Ultimately, she describes herself as pragmatic. It is not that she is unable to consider other options, her current experience is simply how life is. She realizes that she is not thriving at the moment, and is able to consider the danger that her skipped doses may lead to regarding her hypertension, but at the moments when her mood is low she has difficulty motivating herself.

Following a particularly difficult week at work, she has the following discussion in session:

Rebecca: So this week I went in, and someone … I'm assuming my boss again … left a sheet on the printer title "Best Lesbian Jokes of 2019." It was tasteless and degrading, I was so angry.

Therapist: So what did you do?

R: Well, I've given up on trying to talk with HR, they have blown it off as just office humor, and seem uncomfortable with my sexuality. I'm also concerned that if I try and escalate I might get fired, and I'm only putting up with all of this to care for myself.

T: What does your mind tell you about this situation?

R: That I'm in it alone. I've always handled things myself, and I don't have anyone I can turn to.

T: How believable is that thought? The one that says "I have to do this all on my own"?

R: I mean … very believable. It's how my whole life has been.

T: What would you do tomorrow if you woke up and that was unbelievable? If you simply didn't buy it?

R: I'd probably call up a friend and leave, stay on a couch back home or something.

T: What stops you now?

R: People have their own things they're worried about. I have applied for a transfer, I just have to keep applying. No one wants to be put out on my account.

T: What if you didn't believe that thought when you woke up tomorrow? That no one would want to be put out?

R: Oh, then I'd move in a heartbeat back home! I'd call friends until I had a place lined up for a few months and would look for jobs there.

T: It's like these thoughts are heavy weights around your neck, keeping you from moving.

R: Well, they're my reality.

T: Would you be willing to try something? I know that these thoughts are feeling very heavy and believable right now. Would you be willing to wear these thoughts around your neck, weighing you down, and to try and call friends at home at the same time?

R: I'd be embarrassed to do that.

T: Okay, so this is one more thought around your neck, weighing you down. "It would be embarrassing and too hard to deal with if I asked and was told no." Would you be willing to wear that one, too, and to call a friend back home?

R: Okay. I can try this.

While incorporating some themes of willingness that will be explored further in the next chapter, here you have an illustration of externalizing fused thoughts with the metaphor of weights around her neck. The fusion with these thoughts has had the function of restricting her behavior, leading her to not take advantage of her rich network of friends in Minneapolis who might support her while she is subjected to daily microaggressions and overt forms of discrimination that may further impact her ability to cope. Such an interaction could also provide helpful information regarding the utility of this approach with Rebecca. If the use of metaphor and externalization of negative thoughts is helpful in this way and she takes actions to improve her situation, this tactic might be revisited to explore associating her hypertension medication with messages of hope and positive thoughts about her future. Mapping the impact of avoidance and cognitive fusion onto the SORC is depicted in Table 4.1.

The relationship between problematic thoughts and behavior is rooted in fusion with those thoughts. This includes internalized stigma, and those unworkable beliefs that are fueled through contact with anti-SGM bias. This case illustrates how fusion with thoughts associated with hopelessness and isolation can narrow an individual's behaviors in a manner that poses barriers to change. As the following chapters explore more active methods of identifying change behaviors and building up relational networks, it is important to consider the role of acceptance and defusion in creating enough spaciousness to try on new behaviors.

Conclusion

Painful thoughts, including internalized stigma, have an effect upon behavior due to fusion and responding to thoughts as if they are reflective

Table 4.1 SORC of the Function of Avoidance and Cognitive Fusion

Stimulus	Organism	Response	Consequence
Rebecca came out more recently, and experiencing discrimination in the workplace appears to be a novel stressor for which she does not have a ready response.	Rebecca experiences cognitive fusion with a number of pessimistic thoughts.	Passive suicidal ideation. Poor medication adherence. Nondisclosure of her current situation to her support network.	Friends and family are unaware of the extent of Rebecca's current crisis. Increased risk of adverse health consequences.
Rebecca is diagnosed with hypertension, for which she is prescribed medication.	Depressed mood and sad affect. Possible anhedonia. Hopelessness.	Rigid pattern of avoidant coping behaviors.	
Rebecca has recently relocated away from a strong family and friend support network that has not been replaced.			

of external reality. When a particular thought is unworkable for sustaining an SGM client's well-being, then fusion and experiential avoidance work in tandem to restrict active coping or change efforts. The first step toward change comes from accepting the present moment as it is, while working to defuse from those thoughts that are preventing change. Though often associated with mindfulness, both acceptance and defusion may be helpfully considered discreet processes that can target internalized stigma.

Key points

- Internalized stigma can be responded to with acceptance and defusion techniques.
- Acceptance and defusion are key components of psychological flexibility, and may promote behavior change and action through changing a client's relationship with painful thoughts and feelings.
- Defusion is a technique that can only be applied to our relationship with thoughts, not to external events or objects, and should be used alongside acceptance in an affirming manner.

Recommended readings

Blackledge, J. T. (2015). *Cognitive defusion in practice: A clinician's guide to assessing, observing, and supporting change in your client.* New Harbinger Publications.

Skinta, M. D., & D'Alton, P. (2016). Mindfulness and acceptance for malignant shame. In M. D. Skinta and A. Curtin (Eds.). *Mindfulness and acceptance for gender and sexual minorities: A clinician's guide to fostering compassion, connection, and equality using contextual strategies.* New Harbinger Publications.

Stitt, A. (2020). *ACT for gender identity: The comprehensive guide.* Jessica Kingsley Publishers.

References

American Psychological Association (2012). Guidelines for psychological practice with lesbian, gay, and bisexual clients. *American Psychologist*, 67(1), 10-42.

American Psychological Association. (2015). Guidelines for psychological practice with transgender and gender nonconforming people. *American Psychologist*, 70(9), 832–864.

Austin, A., Craig, S. L., & D'Souza, S. A. (2018). An AFFIRMative cognitive behavioral intervention for transgender youth: Preliminary effectiveness. *Professional Psychology: Research and Practice*, 49(1), 1–8.

Aymer, S. R. (2016). "I can't breathe": A case study—Helping Black men cope with race-related trauma stemming from police killing and brutality. *Journal of Human Behavior in the Social Environment*, 26(3–4), 367–376.

Bai, Z., Luo, S., Zhang, L., Wu, S., & Chi, I. (2020). Acceptance and commitment therapy (ACT) to reduce depression: A systematic review and meta-analysis. *Journal of Affective Disorders*, 260, 728–737.

Bhambhani, Y., Flynn, M. K., Kellum, K. K., & Wilson, K. G. (2020). The role of psychological flexibility as a mediator between experienced sexual racism and psychological distress among men of color who have sex with men. *Archives of Sexual Behavior*, 49(2), 711–720.

Blackledge, J. T. (2015). *Cognitive defusion in practice: A clinician's guide to assessing, observing, and supporting change in your client.* New Harbinger Publications.

Bond, F. W., Hayes, S. C., Baer, R. A., Carpenter, K. M., Guenole, N., Orcutt, H. K., ... Zettle, R. D. (2011). Preliminary psychometric properties of the Acceptance and Action Questionnaire–II: A revised measure of psychological inflexibility and experiential avoidance. *Behavior Therapy, 42*(4), 676–688.

Byrne, S. P., Haber, P., Baillie, A., Costa, D. S., Fogliati, V., & Morley, K. (2019). Systematic reviews of mindfulness and acceptance and commitment therapy for alcohol use disorder: Should we be using third wave therapies? *Alcohol and Alcoholism, 54*(2), 159–166.

Dinis, A., Carvalho, S., Gouveia, J. P., & Estanqueiro, C. (2015). Shame memories and depression symptoms: The role of cognitive fusion and experiential avoidance. *International Journal of Psychology and Psychological Therapy, 15*(1), 63–86.

Feliu-Soler, A., Montesinos, F., Gutiérrez-Martínez, O., Scott, W., McCracken, L. M., & Luciano, J. V. (2018). Current status of acceptance and commitment therapy for chronic pain: A narrative review. *Journal of Pain Research, 11*, 2145–2159.

Gilpin, H. R., Stahl, D. R., & McCracken, L. M. (2019). A theoretically guided approach to identifying predictors of treatment outcome in contextual cognitive behavioural therapy for chronic pain. *European Journal of Pain, 23*(2), 354–366.

Hayes, S. C., Strosahl, K. D., & Wilson, K. G. (2011). *Acceptance and Commitment Therapy: The Process and Practice of Mindful Change*, 2nd Edition. Guilford Press.

Lundgren, T., Dahl, J., & Hayes, S. C. (2008). Evaluation of mediators of change in the treatment of epilepsy with acceptance and commitment therapy. *Journal of Behavioral Medicine, 31*(3), 225–235.

Puckett, J. A., & Levitt, H. M. (2015). Internalized stigma within sexual and gender minorities: Change strategies and clinical implications. *Journal of LGBT Issues in Counseling, 9*(4), 329–349.

Reyes-Ortega, M. A., Miranda, E. M., Fresán, A., Vargas, A. N., Barragán, S. C., Robles García, R., & Arango, I. (2019). Clinical efficacy of a combined acceptance and commitment therapy, dialectical behavioural therapy, and functional analytic psychotherapy intervention in patients with borderline personality disorder. *Psychology and Psychotherapy: Theory, Research and Practice*. Advance article online.

Singh, R. S., & O'Brien, W. H. (2020). The impact of work stress on sexual minority employees: Could psychological flexibility be a helpful solution? *Stress and Health, 36*(1), 59–74.

Skinta, M. D., & D'Alton, P. (2016). Mindfulness and acceptance for malignant shame. In M. D. Skinta & A. Curtin (Eds.). *Mindfulness and acceptance for gender and sexual minorities: A clinician's guide to fostering compassion, connection, and equality using contextual strategies.* New Harbinger Publications.

Sloshower, J., Guss, J., Krause, R., Wallace, R. M., Williams, M. T., Reed, S., & Skinta, M. D. (2020). Psilocybin-assisted therapy of major depressive disorder using acceptance and commitment therapy as a therapeutic frame. *Journal of Contextual Behavioral Science, 15,* 12–19.

Skinta, M. D., Lezama, M., Wells, G., & Dilley, J. W. (2015). Acceptance and compassion-based group therapy to reduce HIV stigma. *Cognitive and Behavioral Practice, 22*(4), 481–490.

Stief, M. (2017). The sexual orientation and gender presentation of hijra, kothi, and panthi in Mumbai, India. *Archives of Sexual Behavior, 46*(1), 73–85.

Twohig, M. P., & Levin, M. E. (2017). Acceptance and commitment therapy as a treatment for anxiety and depression: A review. *Psychiatric Clinics, 40*(4), 751–770.

Wharton, E., Edwards, K. S., Juhasz, K., & Walser, R. D. (2019). Acceptance-based interventions in the treatment of PTSD: Group and individual pilot data using acceptance and commitment therapy. *Journal of Contextual Behavioral Science, 14,* 55–64.

Yadavaia, J. E., & Hayes, S. C. (2012). Acceptance and commitment therapy for self-stigma around sexual orientation: A multiple baseline evaluation. *Cognitive and Behavioral Practice, 19*(4), 545–559.

5

VALUES AND COMMITTED ACTION

Introduction

Contingent self-worth, a challenge common across SGM identities, was first known in the literature as the "best little boy in the world" phenomena (Pachankis & Hatzenbuehler, 2013). This gendered designation drew its name from the title of an autobiographical novel, originally published under a pseudonym, by a successful executive and Ivy League graduate who described a life defined by pursuing success in societally approved ways that might allow his family to be proud of and accept him (Tobias, 2010). The general idea resonates with many SGM clients – if I am only good enough, well-behaved enough, and successful enough, I can evade the slings and arrows of those who might mistreat me due to my gender presentation or sexual orientation. Such a stance in life comes with a cost, however. Attending to the greatest desires and expectations of others, or of generic markers of success in society at large, requires a degree of alienation from one's own intrinsic measure of meaningfulness.

One might think of the allure of following a conventional path of success seeking, and the praise it brings, as a loop of positive reinforcement that draws one ever further from attending to one's personal, individual aspirations.

This type of success is a double-edged sword. SGM individuals who experience contingent self-worth may wind up struggling for a sense of meaning, feeling unhappy, and feeling let down with their successes when others do not recognize those efforts. More broadly, they may express difficulty in tacting – the ability to recognize and label those moments that are intrinsically meaningful and to attach a label to those values (Bonow & Follette, 2009). An SGM client will express difficulty choosing a meaningful direction or consider how to define life on their own terms if life has never led to the chance to do so. A value, in this case, can be considered an intrinsically reinforcing direction that elicits a sense of meaning in the client. Unlike a goal, a value is a direction, so when exploring values clarification it may be helpful to share that while a goal can be completed, a value cannot be (Hayes et al., 2011). In introducing the topic of values, I find it helpful to consider the model of behaviors being under appetitive or aversive control. That is, is your client making decisions or choosing their direction in life based upon what they would like to build, or is the choice motivated by avoiding unwanted outcomes? Animal studies in this area suggest that when faced with a moment that contains elements of both, avoidance wins (e.g., Weiss & Schindler, 1989). A real-world example you might consider would be sitting across from the dinner table from your parents while they ask you to open up about your life. This may have served as a prompt for closeness and warmth in the past, though may be competing against an urge to disclose information to which they may respond negatively, such as coming out, or sharing your excitement over a new connection with an affirming medical provider when your parents responded poorly to learning your true gender. In studies with pigeons, that would be where the story ends – no new disclosures are coming for your parents. Human verbal abilities to add meaning to our actions changes all of this, however. This chapter will explore the role of values, techniques on increasing contact with them, and then building from values to committed actions – behavior change intended to bring one's daily life into greater alignment with those values once they have been identified.

Values clarification

It should be noted that while values are being singled out within this chapter as an alternative to contingent self-worth, there is no specific literature on the identification and strengthening of values as an isolated aspect of SGM experiences. Evidence supporting this approach can be derived from three separate areas: pilot studies that include values as a standard piece of ACT interventions with SGM clients, evidence in general populations for values clarification as an effective addition to treatment, and findings on SGM resilience that suggest specific values that may be suggested for consideration by SGM clients. Taken as a collective body of work, values clarification may be a meaningful part of therapy to reduce the impact of minority stress.

Values clarification is most notably a feature in ACT, an experiential, behavioral therapy that emphasizes acceptance processes described in Chapter 4 with values clarification and behavior changes consistent with those values (i.e., committed action; Hayes et al., 2011). In pilot studies with SGM clients, it should be noted that participants across studies are primarily cisgender sexual minorities (e.g., Yadavaia & Hayes, 2012), and skewed toward gay-identified men living with HIV (Moitra et al., 2011; Skinta et al., 2015). Though none of these studies reported specific outcomes regarding values clarification or change as a mechanism of action, participant quotes were noted in one pilot that highlighted the importance of the values component in creating a meaningful life that differed from their experience prior to the intervention (Skinta et al., 2015). Further evidence can be found in ACT research exploring the specific impact of values, though such studies generally consider values within the implementation of ACT that include five other hypothesized mechanisms of action (e.g., Lundgren et al., 2008). In a population living with chronic pain, values-based action within an ACT protocol had a large effect size in post-treatment and follow-up on self-reported symptoms of depression, anxiety, physical disability, and psychological disability (McCracken & Gutiérrez-Martínez, 2011). One study comparing the mechanism of action in ACT and cognitive therapy among clients with anxiety or depression found that willingness to engage in meaningful behaviors in the presence of unwanted emotions and thoughts was supported as a part of both therapies (Forman et al., 2012).

Though not typically framed as a set of values, some sources of resilience that have been identified among SGM individuals lend themselves to this purpose. Though discussed in greater detail in Chapter 7, self-compassion and community connectedness are recurrent themes within SGM resilience literature (e.g., Greene & Britton, 2015; Puckett et al., 2015; Vigna et al., 2018). Both self-compassion and community connectedness bear value-like qualities, as they are both aspirational directions and are not achievable as completable goals. An aspirational value of self-compassion can serve clients as a reminder of the desire to care for themselves in a world full of challenges, just as a value of community may orient a client's attention toward those who are sharing their experience in a challenging moment. In proposing the addition of an aspirational value, it can be helpful to consider the formula of asking permission, providing a rationale, and proposing an action. An example would be, "May I suggest a value I would like to propose adding to your list? [following client assent] There are studies that suggest self-compassion can be an important source of resilience for SGM people. Would you be willing to consider self-compassion as a value to orient toward each day?" This also may not be a fit. A client who resonates with the process of values clarification may not feel that this fits on their list or is a priority in their life. It is worth considering that this degree of discriminating the internal fit of a value and recognizing that it is not a value is an important skill to develop and build from in the movement from values clarification to committed action, and the clinician can continue to model a compassionate stance and community connectedness.

The values card sort

There are a number of clinical tools that have been developed to identify values. It can be helpful in exploring these tasks with a client to be clear that these are provisional aids to explore what is meaningful. A client high in contingent self-worth, for example, may initially choose values that are intended to please me, conform to their self-presentation that pleases their partner or family, or conform to broader societal expectations. The Personal Values Card Sort was first developed as a part of Motivational Interviewing, an approach that also centers bringing attention to the discrepancy between habitual behaviors and values as a lever for change (Miller & Rollnick, 2012; Miller et al., 2001).

The Personal Values Card Sort consists of 83 values labels and the categories of Not Important to Me, Important to Me, and Very Important to Me. There are a few slight variations in administration instructions that can be found, though the process is the same. First, ask the client to sort the values cards among the three categories. When this is complete, remove all but the cards in the Very Important to Me stack, and ask that they select their top five cards from within the set. Though some instructions allow for a lengthier final list, the degree of difficulty in sorting at both stages may offer some insight into the client's difficulty in tacting what feels meaningful, such as difficulty sorting any of the cards as Very Important or as Not Important. After those five primary values are selected, ask the client to describe each with a story or personal definition that would allow you to see it. It can be helpful here to probe for a behavioral descriptor, with questions such as "What would I see you doing from across the street, in passing, that might tell me this is one of your values?" or "Is there a scene in a movie that comes to mind, when someone's actions show they share this value?"

Once there is clarity on what those values are and what behaviors may correspond with those values, it can be helpful to ask the client about the smallest daily behavior they can engage in that would orient them toward that value. Sometimes a client is wrestling with a particular choice, such as coming out to someone or ending a dissatisfying relationship. In these moments, it can be helpful to explore how the client's decision moves them toward or away from each value. Recall that the goal of this task is to increase a client's ability to recognize what feels meaningful, so there are no right or wrong values. Over the course of treatment, some clients will ask to complete the card sort or other values-related tasks again, as their confidence grows in identifying what is more meaningful to them.

Committed action

Values clarification is most beneficial to the degree that it leads to behavior change. As noted earlier in the book, the separate processes explored here often overlap, and committed action is grounded in the acceptance skills explored in Chapter 4. The reason meaningful behaviors may not have been enacted at the time a client enters therapy relate to the aversive control of behavior mentioned earlier in this chapter. When a client's attention is oriented toward environmental threats and interpersonal challenges, effective short-term solutions may undermine engaging in the world in a meaningful way. A bisexual client may value authenticity yet worry that disclosing a bisexual identity could be met with fear, rejection, or assumptions of in-fidelity upon coming out to a spouse or partner who had been unaware of this identity. Choosing, again and again, to not disclose may reduce the likelihood of conflict in the moment, though for the client who finds meaning in feeling authentic and genuine, the long-term trajectory is one of self-alienation and dissatisfaction. For these reasons, it can be helpful to explore with clients what unwanted feelings, emotions, or responses from meaningful others in their life are likely to be encountered if a client changed their behavior to better align with values. This process of choosing values that co-occur with unwanted experiences is labeled *willingness*.

Both ACT and DBT emphasize the role of willingness, which DBT helpfully contrasts with *willfulness* (e.g., Twohig & Peterson, 2009). That is, the goal is not to "push through" or grit one's teeth and endure difficulties. Rather, it is a recognition that unpleasant moments are being chosen be-cause, much like buying a ticket for the subway, the currency of committed action in a valued direction is stamped on the same ticket as painful ex-periences. This is not merely a philosophical stance –SGM individuals who live openly and authentically often have no choice but to experience ex-posure to unasked-for and hateful responses from strangers, or the possi-bility of experiencing discrimination. Practicing willingness involves embracing that a life true to one's values and meaningfully lived involves a loss of control over how others respond and the difficulties inherent within those moments – and remembering that every moment is a new choice. An individual can deeply value authenticity, while simultaneously recognizing that a particular professional or personal context is not welcoming or dangerous and choose to not express themselves in that moment. When approaching the world with open eyes and an awareness of the limitations of the world as it currently exists, choice becomes possible.

The smallest possible step

When working with clients on selecting new behaviors to try through the week, it can be helpful to encourage the smallest possible step. While a client who has felt a lack of meaning in their life may hope that a grand gesture could realign their experience of the world, maintaining an awareness of what is meaningful and what one chooses in each moment is an ongoing, daily task. For instance, when I think of my own experiences choosing to pursue a degree in clinical psychology to promote SGM-sensitive therapies and research, it was already clear to me that this would not always be a positive and supportive experience. While I was fortunate to have many supportive or SGM-identified mentors and supervisors over the years, I was also exposed at every level of training and professional work to individuals who pathologized SGM experiences (both indirectly and clearly), or who expressed discomfort or disdain for more SGM-inclusive stances within the field. Though unaware of values work at that time, at each stage I was motivated by an awareness of how I might more effectively support the community after completing my studies, and the recognition that any painful experiences I encountered were necessary if I were going to reduce the likelihood of SGM students and trainees experiencing such moments in the future.

Case example

Cassie is a 28-year-old transgender White woman who first entered therapy for post-traumatic stress disorder (PTSD) resulting from intimate partner violence in a past relationship with a cisgender man. Cassie has declined exposure-based treatment in the past, though her trauma symptoms have increased in recent months. Her primary symptoms involve intrusive memories and nightmares, though in particular settings or difficult interpersonal exchanges she has recently found herself flooded by certain scenes from the abuse and experiencing panic. This has interfered with her graduate work in social work, as well as her organizing efforts as a part of a regional LGBTQ+ social work organization. At the time she sought treatment, she had begun to skip meetings with her organization's board that she is a member of when she suspected that conflicts may arise, has increasingly missed class, and has begun to isolate herself at home. Relatedly, her activism on campus has led to her being nominated for a student leadership award. Though she has taken estrogen hormone therapy for 6 years and presents as a woman in most areas of her life, she has not told any of her family members. When she attends family events, she does not wear makeup and wears neutral, loose clothing such as sweatshirts and loose-fitting jeans. She is unsure if any of them suspect her gender identity, though no one in her family has commented on any observations. She is concerned that if she allows herself to proceed and receives this recognition from her organization, family members in her community will become aware of her gender identity. Though she has not discussed gender with her family previously, she describes her family as "somewhat traditional," with most men in her family working in stereotypical occupations such as construction or the military, and most women in her family opting between part-time service jobs or homemaking.

In session, Cassie has shared that she sees these concerns related, as she has never disclosed her experience with intimate partner violence to her family – she identifies as heterosexual and does not wish to deal with her family's confusion or be labeled "gay" – and she feels that what was a warm and connected relationship with her family in childhood has been undermined through her limited contact at family events. She also has concerns that if exposure-based therapy for trauma is difficult, she would not have ready access to her emotional support from her family.

At this point, the therapist and Cassie had the following conversation:

Therapist: It feels like we have circled back to this ambivalence for a while. In the card sort, you identified that two of your most important values are family and equality [through activism]. How do these fit together here?

Cassie: This is the problem. I mean, I can't have both, and they're both so important to me. I'm really proud of my activism, but I can't move forward in therapy or take care of myself without my family. I don't know what to do.

T: It sounds like whatever you do, you lose control of what happens next. Right now, if you don't go forward with the award you can control some of your family learning your full identity, and if you choose to proceed in trauma therapy your mind is saying you have to do it without them.

C: Exactly … I wish there were a way that they just wouldn't ask any questions but I could count on them.

T: Is there a version of the future where you never share your identity with them, or your name, and it feels close and connected again?

C: No ... no, I don't think I'd feel that way. I think at some point they'll know and I'll just know for sure which ones care about me and which ones don't accept me.

T: Does this weigh on you now? This idea that when you're speaking with a family member, you don't know which group they're in?

C: All the time! It's one of the reasons I don't attend many family events anymore.

T: What does this do for you? Not telling them?

C: Well, I mean ... I guess I don't have to know for sure. I mean, sure I may be spending time with an aunt or cousin who would reject me, but I also get to hold on to thinking that maybe they'd accept me.

T: So if you wanted to buy a ticket to this future life – to one where you know who you can count on and who may support you, and have support to care for yourself, requires giving up that control? That you can buy a ticket to that life, but the purchase price is no longer holding on to that uncertainty? Is that something you might be willing to do, if this ticket were the only way to move from here to there?

C: I think. ... I think maybe. I'm not sure yet. What's the right choice?

T: Only you know that. For some this would be worth it, and for others it may feel like the ticket is too expensive. You can hold off or buy this ticket at any time. What happens if you choose neither path, like you chose today, and yesterday? What is happening to your relationship with your family?

C: I guess right now we're pretty distant. I feel like I am losing my relationship with my family already.

T: Okay, so that's another option on the table. Not deciding may be a choice to lose them. Choosing to come out may lead to losing or gaining closeness, though there is no way to be certain.

In this case, Cassie has begun to explore willingness, as well as the function of her current decision not to come out to her family. The goal here is not to pressure Cassie that there is a right decision, rather to highlight that there is a decision. Some clients experience such a stark contrast as a surprise, whereas others express relief at considering or reclaiming an active role in a situation that has begun to be experienced as subject to chance and other's actions. Louisa is also experiencing an ongoing refinement of what this value of family means. That is, her responses suggest that while her family is important to her, she also feels disconnected in not knowing who would accept her fully if given the opportunity. A client like Cassie may never decide to disclose, and she may invest in deepening relationships elsewhere in her life for needed support as she begins more active trauma treatment. She also may opt for a partial willingness to lose control. For example, if she were to proceed with the nomination and receive her award, it is possible that some family members may become aware, or none of them. If some family members do become aware, there is a possibility of receiving support from some of them currently as well as support in deciding whether or not to come out to other family members. The SORC depiction of the role that contingent self-worth and values play is illustrated in Table 5.1.

Table 5.1 SORC of the Function of Contingent Self-Worth and Values

Stimulus	Organism	Response	Consequence
Cassie experienced her childhood relationships as warm and loving. Cassie's family is expecting her to meet success and respond to her as a traditional man. Cassie has experienced intimate partner violence in the past. PTSD diagnosis.	Cassie fears that coming out to her family will jeopardize her relationships. Cassie is proud of her in an LGBTQ+ community organization. Cassie's experience of self-worth is contingent on the approval or acceptance of her family. Intrusive thoughts and memories, as well as nightmares. Panic.	Avoidance of situations that might expose her to the direct judgments of her family. Avoidance of conflict. An experience of a values conflict. Deferring painful decisions.	Therapist may feel stuck. Family members experience Cassie as pulling away or guarded.

Using values in this way creates a touchstone for therapy to revisit in the future. If these two values (family and equality) feel unclear in their implementation, there are other values that she might choose to focus on today. This case also illustrates an example of a client who may benefit from considering self-compassion as a value to work toward, as this may encourage her to consider what behaviors she would choose if the primary value were caring for herself in a loving way, cognizant of her own needs. It also appears through an examination of the function of avoiding deciding that she is already growing apart from her family and not benefiting from their support while she decides her next course of action.

Conclusion

Contingent self-worth affects the ability of SGM people to craft meaningful, vibrant lives. Through reorienting to an emphasis on values that allow an SGM person to experience life as meaningful, as well as taking concrete steps toward aligning daily behaviors with those values, clinicians can aid clients in shifting away from contingent self-worth. Willingness to experience the challenges that these actions carry with them, while emphasizing choice in every moment as to whether or not a particular action is worth that cost can promote behavioral flexibility and an awareness that one can do what they can, when they can, without becoming overwhelmed by either a rigid avoidance of bias or an equally rigid standard of behavior.

Key points

- Values are an intrinsically reinforcing orientation toward those factors that make life more meaningful. Committed action refers to those behaviors taken in the service of moving toward values.
- Contingent self-worth among SGM people is exacerbated by anti-SGM environments and the desire to maintain relationships and respect from others.
- Engaging in committed actions that increase the likelihood of exposure to anti-SGM bias requires willingness, or the recognition that valued actions often require the possibility of exposure to pain.

Recommended reading

Dahl, J., Lundgren, T., Plumb, J., & Stewart, I. (2009). *The art and science of valuing in psychotherapy: Helping clients discover, explore, and commit to valued action using acceptance and commitment therapy.* New Harbinger Publications.

Pachankis, J. E., & Hatzenbuehler, M. L. (2013). The social development of contingent self-worth in sexual minority young men: An empirical investigation of the "Best Little Boy in the World" hypothesis. *Basic and Applied Social Psychology, 35*(2), 176–190.

References

Bonow, J. T., & Follette, W. C. (2009). Beyond values clarification: Addressing client values in clinical behavior analysis. *The Behavior Analyst, 32*(1), 69–84.

Forman, E. M., Chapman, J. E., Herbert, J. D., Goetter, E. M., Yuen, E. K., & Moitra, E. (2012). Using session-by-session measurement to compare mechanisms of action for acceptance and commitment therapy and cognitive therapy. *Behavior Therapy, 43*(2), 341–354.

Greene, D. C., & Britton, P. J. (2015). Predicting adult LGBTQ happiness: Impact of childhood affirmation, self-compassion, and personal mastery. *Journal of LGBT Issues in Counseling, 9*(3), 158–179.

Hayes, S. C., Strosahl, K. D., & Wilson, K. G. (2011). *Acceptance and commitment therapy: The process and practice of mindful change* (2nd ed.). Guildford Press.

Lundgren, T., Dahl, J., & Hayes, S. C. (2008). Evaluation of mediators of change in the treatment of epilepsy with acceptance and commitment therapy. *Journal of Behavioral Medicine, 31*(3), 225–235.

McCracken, L. M., & Gutiérrez-Martínez, O. (2011). Processes of change in psychological flexibility in an interdisciplinary group-based treatment for chronic pain based on acceptance and commitment therapy. *Behaviour Research and Therapy, 49*(4), 267–274.

Miller, W. R., C'de Baca, J., Matthews, D. B., & Wilbourne, P. L. (2001). *Personal values card sort.* Albuquerque, NM: University of New Mexico.

Miller, W. R., & Rollnick, S. (2012). *Motivational interviewing: Helping people change.* Guilford Press.

Moitra, E., Herbert, J. D., & Forman, E. M. (2011). Acceptance-based behavior therapy to promote HIV medication adherence. *AIDS Care, 23*(12), 1660–1667.

Pachankis, J. E., & Hatzenbuehler, M. L. (2013). The social development of contingent self-worth in sexual minority young men: An empirical investigation of the "Best Little Boy in the World" hypothesis. *Basic and Applied Social Psychology, 35*(2), 176–190.

Puckett, J. A., Levitt, H. M., Horne, S. G., & Hayes-Skelton, S. A. (2015). Internalized heterosexism and psychological distress: The mediating roles of self-criticism and community connectedness. *Psychology of Sexual Orientation and Gender Diversity, 2*(4), 426–435.

Skinta, M. D., Lezama, M., Wells, G., & Dilley, J. W. (2015). Acceptance and compassion-based group therapy to reduce HIV stigma. *Cognitive and Behavioral Practice, 22*(4), 481–490.

Tobias, A. (2010). *The best little boy in the world grows up.* Ballantine Books.

Twohig, M. P., & Peterson, K. A. (2009). Distress tolerance. In W. T. O'Donohue, & J. E. Fisher, (Eds.). *General principles and empirically supported techniques of cognitive behavior therapy (pp. 265–271).* Hoboken, NJ: John Wiley & Sons, Inc.

Vigna, A. J., Poehlmann-Tynan, J., & Koenig, B. W. (2018). Does self-compassion facilitate resilience to stigma? A school-based study of sexual and gender minority youth. *Mindfulness, 9*(3), 914–924.

Weiss, S. J., & Schindler, C. W. (1989). Integrating control generated by positive and negative reinforcement on an operant baseline: Appetitive-aversive interactions. *Animal Learning & Behavior, 17*(4), 433–446.

Yadavaia, J. E., & Hayes, S. C. (2012). Acceptance and commitment therapy for self-stigma around sexual orientation: A multiple baseline evaluation. *Cognitive and Behavioral Practice, 19*(4), 545–559.

6

VULNERABILITY AND INTIMACY

Introduction

The use of your own authenticity, vulnerability, and warmth as a clinician to effect changes in interpersonal behaviors was introduced in Chapter 2. Specific recommendations and discussions of how this might appear in practice follow, as adopting a therapeutic stance that may be experienced as affirming and caring is only half of the equation. This still requires careful consideration of how and when that warmth is expressed in therapy, and the systematic consideration of the purpose of engaging with your clients in a vulnerable way. Within the spectrum of contextual behavioral therapies, functional analytic psychotherapy (FAP) presents the clearest articulation of how to work within the relationship in a manner that can result in generalizable behavior changes within the client's life (Kohlenberg & Tsai, 1991). In this chapter, rejection sensitivity will specifically be considered as the mechanism most amenable to change through a systematic, process-oriented approach to the use of the therapeutic relationship.

Interpersonal aspects of minority stress

Between internalized stigma and the discriminatory actions of others, minority stress theory has always included midlevel stressors such as rejection sensitivity and self-concealment that reflect an awareness of the bias that exists in the world (Dyar et al., 2018; Hendricks & Testa, 2012). More recent attention has highlighted rejection sensitivity as a specific transdiagnostic psychological risk factor that affects sexual and gender minority (SGM) people and merits greater attention as a site for intervention (Cohen, Feinstein, Rodriguez-Seijas, Taylor, & Newman, 2016; Feinstein, 2019). Parental or familial rejection accounts for much of the variance that has been observed, and rejection sensitivity has been associated with both psychopathology and suicidality (Pachankis, Goldfried, & Ramrattan, 2008; Puckett, Woodward, Mereish, & Pantalone, 2015; Ryan, Huebner, Diaz, & Sanchez, 2009). These experiences of rejection, and the subsequent guardedness that SGM individuals adopt in related to others, have the effect of increasing loneliness and isolation (Mereish & Poteat, 2015). Among gender minority individuals, this interpersonal guardedness may be further fueled by high rates of discrimination, prejudice, and exposure to violent acts (White Hughto, Reisner, & Pachankis, 2015).

One area of research that supports the role of histories of rejection in leading to the development of these patterns can be found in observing the inverse, as SGM youth with supportive parents appear to thrive (Olson, Durwood, DeMeules, & McLaughlin, 2016; Ryan, Russell, Huebner, Diaz, & Sanchez, 2010). There is also evidence that in contexts that allow for relationships to be mended between SGM individuals and rejecting parents, clients experience improvement in their well-being and relationships. Relationship-Focused Therapy for Sexual and Gender Minority Individuals and their Parents (RFT-SGM) is a time-limited, manualized therapy for work with SGM individuals who have been "out" for at least 1 year, though the relationship between parents and an adult child are marked by ongoing tension, conflict, or deterioration of family relationships or family members' well-being (Diamond, Boruchovitz-Zamir, Gat, & Nir-Gottlieb, 2019; Diamond & Shpigel, 2014). Though this chapter emphasizes work with the individual, the effectiveness of RFT-SGM speaks to SGM clients' histories of rejection as a determining factor in developing interpersonal guardedness and relationship difficulties.

A related process leads to the experience of self-concealment, as SGM individuals may seek to minimize risks of harm through reducing their exposure to those who would discriminate against them. Self-concealment efforts may range from a sharp distinction between one's private and public life, attempting to present authentically among friends while avoiding attention within one's professional life, or may be expressed through greater efforts at concealment when the environment is more dangerous (e.g., Sedlovskaya et al., 2013). Among gay men, there is a strong association between concealment and depression, whether observing current concealment or retrospective accounts of having concealed one's identity throughout adolescence (e.g., Frost & Bastone, 2007; Frost et al., 2007). Fortunately, tools have been developed to practice and develop authentic styles of relating within a contextual behavioral framework.

FAP

FAP is a present-moment, behavior analytic approach to enhancing intimacy, genuine responding, and vulnerability in interpersonal relationships. The goals of FAP appear to lend themselves well to the goals of undermining rejection sensitivity and self-concealment among SGM individuals (e.g., Skinta, Hoeflein, Muñoz-Martínez, & Rincón, 2018). The function of rejection sensitivity and self-concealment is ultimately to protect the self from the possibility of interpersonal ruptures and isolation. Through the common SGM experiences described above of parental rejection and possibly years of being aware of one's own identity while unable to disclose it to close others, SGM individuals may develop behavioral repertoires that consist of guardedness, compartmentalization of self-presentation, and inauthentic expressions in environments where threats to the self are not clear.

FAP emphasizes the development of vulnerability, awareness, authenticity, and courage (Tsai et al., 2013). The therapist uses the therapeutic relationship to develop an intense, authentic style of relating while promoting generalization of these skills and risk-taking in the client's outside life. It is important to note that the goal of FAP is not indiscriminate openness and vulnerability with everyone. Similar to processes discussed in prior chapters, such as defusion and acceptance (Chapter 4), one goal of FAP is to orient the individual toward external cues that signal safety and relational reciprocity. For instance, a client may be prompted to consider what traits or non-verbal cues they noticed in the therapist during a vulnerable moment that signaled safety, and how those may relate to behaviors they have observed in others in their life. It is an unfortunate reality that for some SGM individuals, concealment in some contexts may remain necessary. Rather, what is being built upon is flexibility and a greater range. Drawing on my background in clinical health psychology, I have often used the metaphor of the chronically injured knee with clients. As one experiences pain while moving through life, those who experience the most difficulty often begin to restrict their movements further and further from the boundaries where pain might occur, and limit their attempts at movement. Psychotherapy for chronic pain involves orienting to the present moment, signs of comfort that change daily, and a willingness to explore limits when the option is to risk pain in a valued activity or to deprive themselves of meaning. Similarly, individual therapy cannot undo the dangers of a world that still discriminates against and rejects SGM people, though it can orient individuals toward noting those signs and opportunities to live a fuller, more expansive life.

FAP functions primarily through evoking *clinically relevant behaviors* (CRBs) in session, and within the FAP literature utilizes the shorthand of CRB1s to refer to those behaviors that reflect disengagement or blocking closeness, and CRB2s to refer to those behaviors that facilitate closeness and interpersonal intimacy (Haworth et al., 2015; Landes et al., 2013). Research on FAP has supported the role of these techniques in increasing CRB2s, such as emotional expressiveness, among clients in their daily lives outside of session (Lizarazo et al., 2015).

Though explored more fully in Chapter 2, the therapeutic relationship in FAP considers the therapeutic relationship to be a "real" relationship between two people, which is its primary divergence from therapies in psychodynamic traditions that emphasize the role of transference. It is incumbent upon the FAP therapist to be comfortable interacting in a natural manner, and to discover within their own style of relating what behaviors appear to reinforce or punish the responses of each client. In studies that have explored the systematic addition and subtraction of FAP techniques, there is support that the approach itself is associated with changes in the client's interpersonal style of relating (Oshiro et al., 2012).

The five rules

FAP's model is relatively straightforward, though given the attention it requires of the therapist can be difficult to implement and requires some training. At its heart are five rules that guide the therapist's style of interaction with the client. These rules are:

1   Watch for CRBs. The initial learning curve for any therapist following this approach is to identify which behaviors reflect the client's expression of genuineness and vulnerability. These may be imperfect or require shaping, so it is important that the therapist consider what broader types of behavior the client experiences difficulty with.
2   Evoke CRBs. The therapist is unable to reinforce behaviors that reflect closeness without those behaviors being present in-session.
3   Reinforce CRB2s. This is the clinician's primary tool in FAP, and involves responding in a genuine, natural way that warmly reinforces the client's bids for closeness.
4   Observe your impact on the client. Not all clients respond to or appreciate the same level of warmth. For some clients, too much warmth too early may seem inauthentic, or for others may flood them with feelings of overexposure. Reinforcement is defined through the greater likelihood that a behavior is repeated, so allow this to be your guide.
5   Promote generalization. The goal is not that the SGM client and therapist experience a warm and close relationship, though this often occurs in FAP. The goal is that the client take their experiences into the rest of their life.

In implementing these rules, it may be helpful for the therapist to consider the general types of interpersonal challenges that clients bring to therapy. In one study of interpersonal difficulties observed among clients from the general population, five common themes were identified: identifying one's needs and asserting them in a relationship; awareness and responsiveness to receiving and giving feedback; difficulties with recognizing one's own thoughts or emotions; difficulties with feeling close, including personal disclosures; and conflict avoidance (Callaghan, 2006). In a collaborative project with colleagues skilled in providing FAP with SGM clients, we reframed these as: limited or unskilled labeling of emotions or tracking of internal sensations; concealment of emotional responses and avoiding the expression of clear needs; avoidance or self-censoring of thoughts or experiences that emphasize one's gender or sexual identity, such as fears about body image or disclosure of attractions; and social submission, expressed through avoiding disagreement or the assertion of a different perspectives (Skinta et al., 2018).

Daily risk logs

One common practice within FAP used to promote generalization of behavior changes in session is the use of daily emotional risk logs. An emotional risk log emphasizes behaviors that feel risky in the sense that they require greater vulnerability or disclosure than an individual is comfortable with or typically engages in. This activity converges with both the ACT encouragement to practice willingness in the presence of unwanted emotions, or many CFT exercises which require exposure to fears of compassion, though the specific emphasis of a daily risk log is to try a behavior that extends beyond one's typical behavior that give rise to nervousness, fear, or shame. This may include asserting a boundary or saying "no" in a relationship, pausing to note the sensations and truly allow themself to feel love or warmth from another, or making a personal disclosure about their feelings toward another.

In practice, clients are asked to track the behavior daily, with supportive instruction about the benefit of tracking to maintain the behavior. On a scale of one to ten, with one being a behavior barely past one's typical response and a ten being an overwhelming or catastrophic exposure to shame or failure, clients are encouraged to consider targeting a two or three each day. This serves to remind the client that the aspiration is not to revolutionize their behavior today, as such major behaviors would likely both burn out the client quickly and require shaping, but rather to build a habit of engaging courageously within their relationships. Considering the common behavioral targets above, or through functional assessment of the client's history or common challenges brought to session, certain targets could be preselected. Alternately, a client might be encouraged to consider multiple possibilities, and often a pattern emerges based on the client's own report of the risk ratings over the course of a few weeks.

For SGM clients, though there is no source of systematic data collected, there are some clusters of targeted risks I have noticed in clinical practice. For those SGM clients toward the beginning of a process of self-discovery or self-disclosure, risks may involve dressing in a more authentic way to work that expresses their gender, speaking up when misgendered, or sharing their sexual orientation to a loved one. For those who have been out much longer, risks often reflect some degree of allowing others to help or receiving loving behaviors from others, which can feel particularly vulnerable for someone whose interactions had previously been more guarded. Conversely, other popular risks involve disclosing a meaningful or loving gesture with someone in their life. These types of risks center the roles of rejection sensitivity and self-concealment, as they require an SGM person to consider others' warmth as authentic, to engage in their relationships in a way that would allow others to reject them, and to be more transparent about their authentic experience with others.

Case example

Brett is a 32-year-old, cisgender, White grace (a contraction of gray ace, or romantic asexual) gay man who entered therapy with low mood and feelings of loneliness. He had noticed some of his friendships had appeared to drift in recent years, though in general he could not point to any one factor or situation that had led to this. He also felt that his family made efforts to connect more deeply with him, yet he was uncomfortable knowing how to respond. He also recently began a relationship, and though his partner does not identify as asexual, he knew Brett's identity prior to the relationship and has voiced comfort with a relationship that does not center on sex with one another. After the third session, Brett voiced his fear that perhaps his asexuality was not real, and that if he continued to work on his relationships, perhaps he would find that he desired sex more frequently. The therapist gently probed his fears on this matter, and shared that many SGM individuals experience barriers to vulnerability, such as rejection sensitivity. The therapist shared his experience that clients who engage more vulnerably in their relationships have never reported a change in their sexual identities, and there was no literature to suggest that may happen. This is consistent with findings that the primary benefit reported by those who actively seek sexual orientation change efforts, the acceptance of one's experience of their sexuality, should be pursued through affirmative approaches (Flentje, Heck, & Cochran, 2014). Brett and the therapist agreed that they could work in general on exploring the client's closeness in his relationships, and that any intention to change Brett's experience of his sexuality would not be a focus of therapy.

In the second session, the therapist introduced the use of risk logs, and Brett began practicing in his daily life. The specific focus of the risks quickly shifted toward disclosing feelings. Brett shared that he began to notice that a part of his lack of disclosure often involved uncertainty about what he was feeling. In part, he felt it was unfair or would be confusing to others if he shared an emotional experience that he could not fully articulate. Therapy was used both to explore and label emotional experiences as well as to consider ways to describe unclear responses without waiting for them to be perfect. The following exchange occurred after a month of sessions:

Therapist: It's good to see you today, Brett. What would you be most uncomfortable telling me about this week?

Brett: [laughs] We're just jumping right in today, I guess? Well, I did have an experience I wanted to tell you about with my boyfriend.

T: What happened?

B: Well, you know I've been practicing not being sure when I share with others. We have typically slept in separate rooms since he moved in. I told him that I was unsure, and worried it would frustrate him if he wanted to have sex, but that I thought I might like to try cuddling before bed, or even sleeping next to one another.

T: How did he take it?

B: He was super open to the idea, and was willing to try it and promised there wouldn't be any pressure. It was really nice. We cuddled, he didn't try and initiate sex, and said he enjoyed it just as much as I did.

T: Wow, so this is a new part of your relationship that you can experience together?

B: Yes! We haven't cuddled every night – there were a couple nights he worked late and I was already asleep – but it seems like we're a bit closer.

T: It also seems like the part of you that was afraid he would push for sex can trust him a bit more now?

B: Yes! I don't think I'd realized how overcontrolled I had been around him, not sure how much touch was okay.

T: Wow. So this is a pretty major move in the relationship, in terms of feeling genuine and fully seen, and that he accepts and loves you. What was it like, sharing this with me?

B: It's funny – it came to mind first as something scary to share, and it wasn't the topic, as much as your response. I wasn't sure if you'd get that this was a big deal for me, or that I was afraid of how it would pan out.

Note the evocative nature of the opening question (Rule 2), the enthusiastic response to Brett's story (Rule 3), and the therapist checking in on how the client is experiencing the interaction (Rule 4). Rule 1 is present throughout, and Rule 5 is present in the risk logs that led to this session. Brett continued to take risks, both with his partner as well as his friends and family. What began as taking risks that included unclear feedback of uncertainty or discomfort that could not be named became more refined over time. He became better skilled at labeling his emotional experiences as they occurred, and sharing them with those close to him. His experience was that his relationships became better. He did not experience change in his experience of asexuality, though as he continued to discuss and have close friends and his boyfriend respond in warm and accepting ways, he realized that this was not a part of him that needed to change or posed any barriers in those relationships. He is also not alone in this. Though I have not found a study that speaks to this specific question, clients of all sexual orientations or gender identities have asked me, at times, if they might expect their identity to change following therapy, after resolving a traumatic event, or if they learned to be more vulnerable. At times the question is closely linked to cultural messages they have received that pathologize their specific identities, at other times they are repeating a lesson from non-affirming therapy they received in the past. While our sexual orientation and identities are not experienced as rigid or unchanging over the lifespan for some individuals, I am always candid that I am unaware of therapies that facilitate this process. I encourage clients to notice their own awareness of their identity as it unfolds in genuine, vulnerable relationships. Mapping the role of rejection sensitivity and identity concealment on the SORC appears in Table 6.1.

Rejection sensitivity and identity concealment create a difficult cycle to break out of. Others may view an SGM individual struggling with rejection sensitivity as timid, unopinionated, or distant. An SGM individual high in

Table 6.1 SORC of the Function of Rejection Sensitivity and Self-Concealment

Stimulus	Organism	Response	Consequence
Brett began treatment open with his family and friends that he was gay, though more selectively open about identifying as asexual. Brett experiences his social network as loose and distant. Brett is in a new relationship.	Brett has some thoughts pathologizing his experience, both his lack of emotional clarity and his identity as asexual. Loneliness. Fears of others rejecting him if he is more open. Brett fears his boyfriend does not really accept his ace identity.	Brett does not disclose his opinions or emotions until he is certain what they are. Brett avoids too much physical contact with his boyfriend, so that he does not need to decline sex.	Friends experience Brett as aloof and independent. They are unlikely to assume he would like to grow closer. Others may view him as mercurial or closed off, with only occasional disclosures of preference. Others may assume he does not hold strong opinions, and fail to ask his views.

pliance and attuned to social rules may also be high in rejection sensitivity, appear to others as affable and open, yet suffer from an inner life that is experienced as ingenuine and disconnected. This case also highlights how broad, societal messages that suggest SGM identities are a result of psychopathology lead some SGM individuals to question if this is true, particularly if they are experiencing challenges elsewhere in life. Through following the principles outlined above to reinforce and strengthen self-awareness and risk taking, clients can better express their most genuine, authentic self with others.

Conclusion

Vulnerability and self-concealment interfere with SGM individual's relationships with others, as well as their relationship with themselves. These habitual patterns undermine meaningful relationships, and it can be difficult to initiate changes in how we behave with others without a warm, receptive person who values those disclosures and the subsequent experience of closeness. When a therapist is able to use their own genuine responses and relationships as a means of reinforcing and supporting those changes, new behaviors are able to take root. As described in part in Chapter 2, engaging in therapy in a manner in which you are experienced as vulnerable, authentic, and genuine by your clients is a prerequisite to conducting this form of interpersonal therapy.

Key points

- Rejection sensitivity and self-concealment contribute to challenges in relationships.
- FAP requires the therapist use their own genuine responses as a key tool in therapy. The therapist must be comfortable staying present with shame, pain, and loss.
- The goal of FAP is to increase authentic, intimacy-oriented behaviors that will be naturally reinforced in the client's life.

Recommended reading

Holman, G., Kanter, J. W., Tsai, M., & Kohlenberg, R. (2017). *Functional analytic psychotherapy made simple: A practical guide to therapeutic relationships*. New Harbinger Publications.

Kohelnerg, R. J., & Tsai, M. (1991). *Functional analytic psychotherapy: Creating intense and curative relationships*. Plenum Press.

Packenham, K. (2020). *The trauma banquet: Eating pain – feasting on life*. Moshpit Publishing.

References

Callaghan, G. M. (2006). The functional idiographic assessment template (FIAT) system: For use with interpersonally-based interventions including functional analytic psychotherapy (FAP) and FAP-enhanced treatments. *The Behavior Analyst Today, 7*, 357–398.

Cohen, J. M., Feinstein, B. A., Rodriguez-Seijas, C., Taylor, C. B., & Newman, M. G. (2016). Rejection sensitivity as a transdiagnostic risk factor for internalizing psychopathology among gay and bisexual men. *Psychology of Sexual Orientation and Gender Diversity, 3*, 259–264.

Diamond, G. M., Boruchovitz-Zamir, R., Gat, I., & Nir-Gottlieb, O. (2019). Relationship-focused therapy for sexual and gender minority individuals and their parents. In J. E. Pachankis & S. A. Safren (Eds.), *Handbook of evidence-based mental health practice with sexual and gender minorities* (pp. 430–456). New York, NY: Oxford University Press.

Diamond, G. M., & Shpigel, M. S. (2014). Attachment-based family therapy for lesbian and gay young adults and their persistently nonaccepting parents. *Professional Psychology: Research and Practice, 45*(4), 258–268.

Dyar, C., Feinstein, B. A., Eaton, N. R., & London, B. (2018). The mediating roles of rejection sensitivity and proximal stress in the association between discrimination and internalizing symptoms among sexual minority women. *Archives of Sexual Behavior, 47*(1), 205–218.

Feinstein, B. A. (2019). The rejection sensitivity model as a framework for understanding sexual minority mental health. *Archives of Sexual Behavior.* Advance article online. https://doi.org/10.1007/s10508-019-1428-3.

Flentje, A., Heck, N. C., & Cochran, B. N. (2014). Experiences of ex-ex-gay individuals in sexual reorientation therapy: Reasons for seeking treatment, perceived helpfulness and harmfulness of treatment, and post-treatment identification. *Journal of Homosexuality, 61,* 1242–1268.

Frost, D. M., & Bastone, L. M. (2007). The role of stigma concealment in the retrospective high school experiences of gay, lesbian, and bisexual individuals. *Journal of LGBT Youth, 5,* 27–36.

Frost, D. M., Parsons, J. T., & Nanín, J. E. (2007). Stigma, concealment and symptoms of depression as explanations for sexually transmitted infections among gay men. *Journal of Health Psychology, 12,* 636–640.

Haworth, K., Kanter, J. W., Tsai, M., Kuczynski, A. M., Rae, J. R., & Kohlenberg, R. J. (2015). Reinforcement matters: A preliminary, laboratory-based component-process analysis of Functional Analytic Psychotherapy's model of social connection. *Journal of Contextual Behavioral Science, 4,* 281–291.

Hendricks, M. L., & Testa, R. J. (2012). A conceptual framework for clinical work with transgender and gender nonconforming clients: An adaptation of the Minority Stress Model. *Professional Psychology: Research and Practice, 43,* 460–467.

Holman, G., Kanter, J. W., Tsai, M., & Kohlenberg, R. (2017). *Functional analytic psychotherapy made simple: A practical guide to therapeutic relationships.* New Harbinger Publications.

Kohlenberg, R. J., & Tsai, M. (1991). *Functional analytic psychotherapy: Creating intense and curative relationships.* Plenum Press.

Landes, S. L., Kanter, J. W., Weeks, C. E., & Busch, A. M. (2013). The impact of the active components of functional analytic psychotherapy on idiographic target behaviors. *Journal of Contextual Behavioral Science, 2,* 49–57.

Lizarazo, N. E., Munoz-Martinez, A. M., Santos, M. M., & Kanter, J. W. (2015). A within-subjects evaluation of the effects of functional analytic psychotherapy on in-session and out-of-session client behavior. *The Psychological Record, 65,* 463–474.

Mereish, E. H., & Poteat, V. P. (2015). A relational model of sexual minority mental and physical health: The negative effects of shame on relationships, loneliness, and health. *Journal of Counseling Psychology, 62,* 425–437.

Olson, K. R., Durwood, L., DeMeules, M., & McLaughlin, K. A. (2016). Mental health of transgender children who are supported in their identities. *Pediatrics, 137,* e20153223. http://dx.doi.org/10.1542/peds.2015-3223.

Oshiro, C. K. B., Kanter, J., & Meyer, S. B. (2012). A single-case experimental demonstration of functional analytic psychotherapy with two clients with severe interpersonal problems. *International Journal of Behavioral and Consultation Therapy, 7,* 111–116.

Pachankis, J. E., Goldfried, M. R., & Ramrattan, M. E. (2008). Extension of the rejection sensitivity construct to the interpersonal functioning of gay men. *Journal of Consulting and Clinical Psychology, 76,* 306–317.

Packenham, K. (2020). *The trauma banquet: Eating pain – feasting on life.* Moshpit Publishing.

Puckett, J. A., Woodward, E. N., Mereish, E. H., & Pantalone, D. W. (2015). Parental rejection following sexual orientation disclosure: Impact on internalized homophobia, social support, and mental health. *LGBT Health, 2,* 265–269.

Ryan, C., Huebner, D., Diaz, R. M., & Sanchez, J. (2009). Family rejection as a predictor of negative health outcomes in white and Latino lesbian, gay, and bisexual young adults. *Pediatrics, 123,* 346–352.

Ryan, C., Russell, S. T., Huebner, D., Diaz, R., & Sanchez, J. (2010). Family acceptance in adolescence and the health of LGBT young adults. *Journal of Child and Adolescent Psychiatric Nursing, 23,* 205–213.

Sedlovskaya, A., Purdie-Vaughns, V., Eibach, R. P., LaFrance, M., Romero-Canyas, R., & Camp, N. P. (2013). Internalizing the closet: Concealment heightens the cognitive distinction between public and private selves. *Journal of Personality and Social Psychology, 104,* 695–715.

Skinta, M. D., Hoeflein, B., Muñoz-Martínez, A. M., & Rincón, C. L. (2018). Responding to gender and sexual minority stress with functional analytic psychotherapy. *Psychotherapy, 55*(1), 63–72.

Tsai, M., Callaghan, G. M., & Kohlenberg, R. J. (2013). The use of awareness, courage, therapeutic love, and behavioral interpretation in Functional Analytic Psychotherapy. *Psychotherapy, 50,* 366–370.

White Hughto, J. M., Reisner, S. L., & Pachankis, J. E. (2015). Transgender stigma and health: A critical review of stigma determinants, mechanisms, and interventions. *Social Science and Medicine, 147,* 222–231.

7

COMPASSION AND COMMUNITY

Introduction

SGM identities are still widely pathologized in the world, with many of those forms of pathologization carrying the message that there is something wrong with SGM individuals that renders them outside of society. Whether through the specter of stranger violence, mistreatment by a medical provider, or the striking loss of contact with one's family following parental rejection, all of these manifestations undermine a sense of safety in the world. One cannot always anticipate the shock of microaggressions within relationships where they are not expected, such as from colleagues or friends. When these instances occur frequently, a likely result is concealment or some degree of constant interpersonal guardedness. Shame, the affective response to a self that seems unlovable or unwanted, undermines an inner sense of safety even when alone (Boehm, 2012). As Dr. Gary Diamond, who has extended attachment-based family therapy to work with reconciling families that rejected SGM children, once noted that, deep down, everyone wants to believe that somewhere out there in the world their mother loves them (Diamond, 2018). In this chapter, we'll be exploring the challenges of shame as well as the resilience that comes from a cultivation of self-compassion and connections within the community.

Shame versus compassion

Shame is described as a *self-conscious* emotion – shame requires both a sense of self and some degree of perspective-taking of other's experiences to develop (e.g., Misailidi, 2020). Many theorists have noted the evolutionary origins and adaptive benefit of shame in a social species like humans (Boehm, 2012). Shame may be considered as a response to signs that we have endangered our standing or acceptance within our particular local social groups, the experience of feeling overexposed and vulnerable, and a desire to hide (e.g., Lindsay-Hartz, 1984). Neurological studies, for example, have noted activation in the same region following social exclusion as is activated during acute physical pain (Eisenberger, 2012), speaking to the likely biological substrate supporting the need for connection among social animals like ourselves.

Compassion, however, might be considered a form of opposite action to shame (e.g., Rizvi & Linehan, 2005). Where shame orients the individual to look inward, overwhelmed by pain in the moment and self-critically assuming this pain is deserved, compassion, particularly self-compassion, encourages the consideration that such pain is human, connects the one experiencing it with others, and promotes the desire to remove that pain in some way. Though some debate exists regarding how best to operationalize compassion, most definitions include some combination of an awareness of other's suffering, empathy or concern for the one suffering, a desire that this suffering be relieved, and a motivation or willingness to take actions that will relieve that suffering (e.g., Jazaieri et al., 2013). Compassion research has flourished over the past decade, leading to the development of compassion-focused therapy (CFT; Gilbert, 2014), as well as a number of psychoeducational training groups, often offered by paraprofessionals. Generally following the model of MBSR described in Chapter 5, these 2-hour, 8- or 9-week courses include Cognitively Based Compassion Training (Pace et al., 2009), Mindful Self-Compassion (Neff & Germer, 2013), Compassion Cultivation Training

(Jazaieri et al., 2013), Cultivating Emotional Balance (Kemeny et al., 2012), Compassion and Loving-Kindness Meditations (e.g., Hoffmann et al., 2011), and Mindfulness-Based Compassionate Living (Schuling et al., 2016).

SGM experiences of shame support its role in undermining the well-being of SGM people. Differences have been found in the association of shame, chronic depression, and early life relationships with parents among gay men (Matos et al., 2017), and a relationship between shame and suicidality across sexual minority identities (Mereish et al., 2019). Though shame is not specifically assessed, exposure to gender identity change efforts, which treat one's gendered self as an unacceptable part of the self, has been associated with adult suicidality among gender minority individuals (Turban et al., 2020).

The literature supporting the effectiveness or efficacy of compassion and self-compassion trainings has not tracked or reported data on SGM participants. This is not uncommon, as few studies that are not specific to the needs of SGM people collect demographic information on gender identity or sexual orientation (e.g., Heck et al., 2017). Existing literature supporting compassion-based interventions are primarily descriptions of proposed interventions (e.g., Pepping et al., 2017) or clinical experience (e.g., Petrocchi et al., 2016). This is an important area of consideration, as self-compassion does appear to be amenable to change, and changes in one's degree of self-compassion appear to result in changes to one's psychological well-being (e.g., Neff et al., 2007). Correlational studies of self-compassion have supported its role as a resilience factor for SGM people. Self-compassion is associated with resilience against psychological distress among SGM youth, including SGM youth of color (Vigna et al., 2018; 2020). Self-compassion also appears to support sexual minority quality of life (Fredrick, LaDuke, & Williams, 2020).

Community connectedness

As this chapter has considered from different perspectives, shame and self-criticism are ameliorated through social safety. There has been some research into SGM individuals more broadly feeling a sense of belonging in their community. Attempts to measure community connection are challenged by differences in race and wealth among those who might feel that local SGM spaces exist for people like them (e.g., Barrett & Pollack, 2005; Han, 2007). Historically, SGM communities have also emphasized the role of *chosen family*, reflecting the construction of networks of mutual support when biological family members reject SGM individuals (e.g., Duran & Pérez, 2019; Muraco, 2006). It is also important to consider expressions of chosen family unique to Black and Latinx communities, such as the ballroom and house families, and combine both a family as well as a larger community network (e.g., Young et al., 2017). The newness of marriage equality means that it is unclear if the historical socio-legal support for a traditional definition of family will ultimately undermine the role of chosen families. There is some data to suggest that the chosen family members still play an important role in the lives of SGM people, even as support grows among biological family members and as opportunities to marry become available (Hull & Ortyl, 2019).

While clients can be encouraged to engage socially, both generally and within the SGM community, this recommendation is deceptive in its simplicity. Clients avoid connecting with their local communities for a variety of reasons, ranging from social anxiety or identity concealment to fears of having negative beliefs confirmed about either the SGM community or themselves. For some clients I have worked with, particularly for those among migrant communities of color seeking to explore community gatherings, there may be fear that their own experience has been too unique and the local community will not be one they see themselves in. In a popular measure of self-compassion (i.e., Self-Compassion Scale; Neff, 2003), this is captured in the conflict between isolation and a sense of common humanity. This is the difference between considering one's sources of pain and suffering as unique events that separate an individual from the rest of humanity, or as shared experiences that connect us all. For those who express a great deal of fear about exploring the local SGM community or a specific community within it that matches their multiple identities, there are a number of interventions that may be helpful. These may include defusion from beliefs about the community (Chapter 4), disclosure by the therapist about the experience of community spaces, or could incorporate perspective-taking through bibliotherapy with books written by authors who share their identities with the client (e.g., Langroudi & Skinta, 2019).

CFT

CFT is the primary expression of how compassion may be used to respond to shame in individual psychotherapy (Gilbert, 2014). CFT draws on the neurophysiology of three motivational systems: threat, drive, and soothing. Often therapy begins with psychoeducation regarding these three systems, their function, and how they interrelate. For instance, I have often asked clients to consider that they begin to learn threat shortly after birth the first time they experience the shock of cold after birth or are startled by a loud noise. The drive, or reward, system begins to be trained the moment a child first tastes milk when hungry. Learning the soothing system through the desire for connectedness and safety is where training may be less consistently automatic. As long as one is alive, experiences of threat or reward (through sating hunger or thirst) are possible, yet there is no guarantee that parents or caretakers are loving, responsive, or supportive.

The result of this is that when one has a less developed soothing system, strong emotional responses are mitigated by drive or threat systems. Life feels good while success is happening, regardless of the lack of social safety in the soothing system. This model parallels the experience of contingent self-worth described in Chapter 5, which also involves a focus on success over feelings of authenticity and intimacy within a relationship.

The social sun

There are as many ways to promote connection and compassion as there are means of connecting as humans. From modified thought records to meditation, any activity that balances exposure to fears of giving or receiving compassion combined with a willingness to be vulnerable in that moment can facilitate growth in the soothing system. One example is the compassionate other meditation, the visualization of an idealized wise and compassionate other, real or fictional, that functions as imaginal exposure to the fear of receiving compassion (e.g., Gilbert, 2010). Another example may be the emotional risk logs described in Chapter 6, as many interpersonal risks require contact with fear of giving or receiving compassion, to self or others.

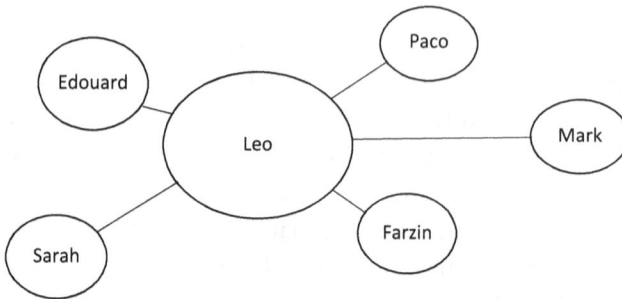

Figure 7.1 Social Sun. After the relationships are mapped, vulnerable attempts to extend warmth to others is added.

The exercise described here is an adaptation of the "social map" exercise from the ERASE-STRESS program, an intervention designed to work with those who have experienced trauma (Berger, 2014). This modification was made with the intention of identifying interpersonal risks that require giving or receiving warmth from another. Given the shape formed by this mapping exercise and the emphasis on finding ways to practice giving warmth to others, this exercise is titled the "social sun."

Clients are asked to begin by drawing a circle and writing their name in the center. Surrounding this circle, they should consider the five to ten most meaningful relationships in their life, and write those names in circles with the distance from the center based upon how close they feel with each person. An example can be seen in Figure 7.1.

After completing this map of close relationships, a client is asked to reflect on those relative distances, and whether any of those lines is further away than they would like it to be. The clinician should explore with the client what specific action the client would be willing to take that they believe would increase the closeness within this relationship. For some clients, fear of lack of reciprocity has led to a pattern of waiting for others to contact them first. For others, a challenging interaction that may have required giving or asking for forgiveness may also have served as a barrier to connection. The social sun exercise allows a client to reflect on how fears of giving or receiving compassion may have functioned to hold others at a distance, and how leaning into those fears may allow a client to increase their experience of contentedness and social safety.

Case example

Rakib is a 24-year-old cisgender gay man from Bangladesh who entered therapy to assist himself in finding greater self-acceptance. He first realized his sexual orientation as an adolescent, attracted to classmates, and as a member of an upper middle-class family he had a relative degree of privacy and freedom to search the internet for information and even to experiment with a classmate once when home alone. His parents discovered his browsing history when he was 16, which led to him being entered into a program that offered sexual orientation change efforts. His parents believed he was "cured" at this time, and after receiving a scholarship to attend a prestigious university in the United States, he remained for graduate school, pursuing a doctoral degree in the field of biology. Rakib was uncomfortable fully disclosing the activities that the sexual orientation change effort involved, though described a great deal of self-isolation and a lingering sense that there was something evil about him that led to him experiencing attraction to other men. He described a split between his mind and his heart, knowing logically that his sexuality was a natural expression of human diversity, yet feeling overwhelming shame when memories of messages that were repeated to him in his childhood arose.

He reported particular difficulty in attempting not to feel that shame and express himself in a free and sexual way. This led to a period of difficulty the year prior with the use of crystal methamphetamine ("meth") during sex. He reported that using meth had allowed him to feel disinhibited and enjoy himself more fully, though the contrast with shameful memories and thoughts that returned while not using had worsened those experiences. At one point, he almost failed a semester of courses in his graduate program, which would have jeopardized his visa and his ability to remain in the United States. Similarly, he had fears that if he relapsed and was arrested with drugs in his possession, this would preclude his ability to seek asylum if he chose to do so at a later time. He reported ongoing challenges with self-critical thoughts and experiencing shame.

In session, therapy has begun to focus on Rakib's experience of "shame spirals" – moments when he experienced a failure in his work or was rejected on a dating app, which led to a cycle of ruminating about his unlovability and self-critical thoughts. A session at this point covered the following dialogues:

Rakib: I was walking past a park the other day and saw a guy I'd hooked up with at a party when I was using. I was just thinking about how my parents would feel if they saw me like that, and kept thinking that was going to be my fate, anyway.

Therapist: What happens when your mind begins going in this direction? What were you feeling after that crossed your mind?

R: It was the same old thing. I couldn't meet anyone's eyes as I walked home, and just wanted to cry. I don't know what makes anything worth it.

                [*After assessing current suicidality, and determining Rakib did not seem to currently be at risk of taking action to harm himself, the session continues …*]

T: What did you do with yourself for the rest of the night?

R: First I got on the apps for a bit. I thought I might find someone to cheer me up. After a while, and not finding anyone, I just drank a few shots and went to bed. I was just trying to shut the day off.

T: If I were telling you about your own best friend, who had been experiencing a difficult day, going home and spending his evening on the apps and then, feeling lonely, drinking a few shots quickly to help fall asleep, what would you say?

R: I mean, I'd feel bad for him and try and cheer him up. I just can't do that for myself.

T: What would you do for him, though? If you were there in that moment remembering how human this is, and how deserving he is of care?

R: might have taken a hot shower after I got home. My coworker in the lab has been trying to be friends and offered to get together for dinner. I might have called him to see what he was doing.

T: How do you think your night would have ended if that had happened last night?

R: I'd have probably not felt so terrible. I'd have maybe even had a nice phone call with my coworker if we didn't get together.

T: What would caring for yourself look like tonight?

R: There's a Trikone meet-up going on tonight [*Trikone is an international non-profit that provides social and political support to LGBT people of South Asian descent*]. I have been meaning to go, so can go tonight?

T: That sounds like it could be a nice way to treat yourself.

There are a few layers here that you might consider. One is the use of perspective-taking – imagining a friend – as a means of considering the sort of treatment that would be beneficial for one's self. Similar strategies of imagining the self through another's eyes or as a stranger are used across compassion interventions to contrast how an individual who experiences a great deal of difficulty receiving compassion or giving it to themself might expect others to be treated. Rakib is able to note the function that his self-criticism and experience of shame play in not caring for himself. He also notes a contrast with how he expects others to be treated, and expresses some willingness to treat himself differently. Working with a client with a strong history of shame and self-criticism, I would emphasize warm encouragement while leaving room for him to experience difficulty following through. Often working with clients high in shame involves a number of gradual approximations and a risk that raising expectations too high begins to be experienced as increasing a likelihood of criticism from the therapist. For example, if Rakib attends the Trikone meeting, he may experience moments of connection and familiarity with other SGM Bangladeshi individuals that feel warm and connecting. He also may feel he does not fit and leave feeling increasingly self-critical, or may not attend and fear disappointing the therapist. All of these outcomes involve an opportunity for the therapist to encourage self-compassion in the following session. The SORC depiction of the role that shame, self-compassion, and community play is illustrated in Table 7.1.

Conclusion

Compassion and connecting with others are deeply interrelated processes according to current theories that underlie CFT (Gilbert, 2014). In a world where SGM identities are pathologized and rejected,

Table 7.1 SORC of the Function of Shame and Self-Criticism.

Stimulus	Organism	Response	Consequence
Rakib has had a traumatic sexual orientation change effort experience that was deeply shaming and pathologizing.	Rakib experiences a deep sense of shame in moments of rejection.	Use of meth. Rumination. Staying at home, not attending community or social events. Declining efforts to connect by coworkers.	Others may feel rejected by Rakib's frequently declining invitations. May appear distant or aloof to others.
Rakib's family now believes him to be heterosexual.	Rakib has recurrent thoughts about something being wrong with him.		
Past substance use, and a visa that could be jeopardized by substance use.	Cravings to use substances when feeling overwhelmed.		

responding with self-criticism or feeling shame about one's identity may be common responses, particularly for those whose histories have not included acceptance. High shame and self-criticism undermines relationships and community with others, connections in interpersonal relationships, and even a sense of contentedness when alone. The combination of working to soothe shame with self-compassion skills and facilitate a sense of belonging in the world through social connection with the broader SGM community may mitigate shame. A willingness to feel and experience the fear of connecting with others while continuing to extend one's self vulnerably play an important part in this work.

Key points

- Societal messages that suggest something is wrong with SGM identities promote shame and self-criticism.
- Self-compassion requires behaving in an opposite manner to shame, and may soothe those experiences.
- Community connectedness supports a sense of belonging in the world, and may further reduce a sense of isolation that undermines self-compassion.

Recommended reading

Germer, C. (2009). *The mindful path to self-compassion: Freeing yourself from destructive thoughts and emotions.* Guilford Press.

Smith, J. G., & Han, C. W. (2019). *Home and community for queer men of color: The intersection of race and sexuality.* Lexington Books.

Tirch, D., Schoendorff, B., & Silberstein, L. R. (2014). *The ACT practitioner's guide to the science of compassion: Tools for fostering psychological flexibility.* New Harbinger Publications.

References

Barrett, D. C., & Pollack, L. M. (2005). Whose gay community? Social class, sexual self-expression, and gay community involvement. *The Sociological Quarterly, 46*(3), 437–456.

Berger, R. (2014). The ERASE-STRESS (ES) programs: A teacher-delivered universal school-based programs in the aftermath of disasters. In D. Mitchel, & V. Karr (Eds.). *Crises, conflict and disability: Ensuring equality.* UK: Routledge.

Boehm, C. (2012). *Moral origins: The evolution of virtue, altruism, and shame.* Basic Books.

Diamond, G. (2018, June). Chair. Promoting healthy sexual behavior, depression and co-occurring alcohol dependence, and psychoanalytic treatment among LGBT individuals. *Symposium presented at the annual convention of the Society for Psychotherapy Research,* Amsterdam, Netherlands.

Duran, A., & Pérez II, D. (2019). The multiple roles of chosen familia: Exploring the interconnections of queer Latino men's community cultural wealth. *International Journal of Qualitative Studies in Education, 32*(1), 67–84.

Eisenberger, N. I. (2012). The neural bases of social pain: Evidence for shared representations with physical pain. *Psychosomatic Medicine, 74*(2), 126–135.

Fredrick, E. G., LaDuke, S. L., & Williams, S. L. (2020). Sexual minority quality of life: The indirect effect of public stigma through self-compassion, authenticity, and internalized stigma. *Stigma and Health, 5*(1), 79–82.

Gilbert, P. (2010). *Compassion focused therapy: Distinctive features.* London, UK: Routledge.

Gilbert, P. (2014). The origins and nature of compassion focused therapy. *British Journal of Clinical Psychology, 53*(1), 6–41.

Han, C. S. (2007). They don't want to cruise your type: Gay men of color and the racial politics of exclusion. *Social Identities, 13*(1), 51–67.

Heck, N. C., Mirabito, L. A., LeMaire, K., Livingston, N. A., & Flentje, A. (2017). Omitted data in randomized controlled trials for anxiety and depression: A systematic review of the inclusion of sexual orientation and gender identity. *Journal of Consulting and Clinical Psychology, 85*(1), 72–76.

Hoffmann, S. G., Grossman, P., & Hinton, D. E. (2011). Loving-kindness and compassion meditation: Potential for psychological intervention. *Clinical Psychology Review, 13*, 1126–1132.

Hull, K. E., & Ortyl, T. A. (2019). Conventional and cutting-edge: Definitions of family in LGBT communities. *Sexuality Research and Social Policy, 16*(1), 31–43.

Jazaieri, H., Jinpa, G. T., McGonigal, K., Rosenberg, E. L., Finkelstein, J., Simon-Thomas, E., & Goldin, P. R. (2013). Enhancing compassion: A randomized controlled trial of a compassion cultivation training program. *Journal of Happiness Studies, 14*(4), 1113–1126.

Kemeny, M. E., Foltz, C., Cavanagh, J. F., Cullen, M., Giese-Davis, J., Jennings, P., ... Ekman, P. (2012). Contemplative/emotion training reduces negative emotional behavior and promotes prosocial responses. *Emotion, 12*, 338–350.

Langroudi, K. F., & Skinta, M. D. (2019). Working with gender and sexual minorities in the context of Islamic culture: A queer Muslim behavioural approach. *The Cognitive Behaviour Therapist, 12*(e21), 1–12.

Lindsay-Hartz, J. (1984). Contrasting experiences of shame and guilt. *American Behavioral Scientist, 27*(6), 689–704.

Matos, M., Carvalho, S. A., Cunha, M., Galhardo, A., & Sepodes, C. (2017). Psychological flexibility and self-compassion in gay and heterosexual men: How they relate to childhood memories, shame, and depressive symptoms. *Journal of LGBT Issues in Counseling, 11*(2), 88–105.

Mereish, E. H., Peters, J. R., & Yen, S. (2019). Minority stress and relational mechanisms of suicide among sexual minorities: Subgroup differences in the associations between heterosexist victimization, shame, rejection sensitivity, and suicide risk. *Suicide and Life-Threatening Behavior, 49*(2), 547–560.

Misailidi, P. (2020). Understanding internal and external shame in childhood: The role of theory of mind. *European Journal of Developmental Psychology, 17*(1), 19–36.

Muraco, A. (2006). Intentional families: Fictive kin ties between cross-gender, different sexual orientation friends. *Journal of Marriage and Family, 68*(5), 1313–1325.

Neff, K. D. (2003). The development and validation of a scale to measure self-compassion. *Self and Identity*, 2(3), (223– 250).

Neff, K. D., & Germer, C. K. (2013). A pilot study and randomized controlled trial of the mindful self-compassion program. *Journal of Clinical Psychology*, 69, 28–44.

Neff, K. D., Kirkpatrick, K. L., & Rude, S. S. (2007). Self-compassion and adaptive psychological functioning. *Journal of Research In Personality*, 41(1), 139–154.

Pace, T. W., Negi, L. T., Adame, D. D., Cole, S. P., Sivilli, T. I., Brown, T. D., … Raison, C. L. (2009). Effect of compassion meditation on neuroendocrine, innate immune and behavioral responses to psychosocial stress. *Psychoneuroendocrinology*, 34(1), 87–98.

Pepping, C. A., Lyons, A., McNair, R., Kirby, J. N., Petrocchi, N., & Gilbert, P. (2017). A tailored compassion-focused therapy program for sexual minority young adults with depressive symptomatology: Study protocol for a randomized controlled trial. *BMC Psychology*, 5(1), 5.

Petrocchi, N., Matos, M., Carvalho, S., & Baiocco, R. (2016). Compassion-focused therapy in the treatment of shame-based difficulties in gender and sexual minorities. In M. D. Skinta and A. Curtin (Eds.). *Mindfulness and acceptance for gender and sexual minorities: A clinician's guide to fostering compassion, connection, and equality using contextual strategies*. Oakland, CA: Context Press.

Rizvi, S. L., & Linehan, M. M. (2005). The treatment of maladaptive shame in borderline personality disorder: A pilot study of "opposite action". *Cognitive and Behavioral Practice*, 12(4), 437–447.

Schuling, R., Huijbers, M. J., van Ravesteijn, H., Donders, R., Kuyken, W., & Speckens, A. E. (2016). A parallel-group, randomized controlled trial into the effectiveness of mindfulness-based compassionate living (MBCL) compared to treatment-as-usual in recurrent depression: Trial design and protocol. *Contemporary Clinical Trials*, 50, 77–83.

Turban, J. L., Beckwith, N., Reisner, S. L., & Keuroghlian, A. S. (2020). Association between recalled exposure to gender identity conversion efforts and psychological distress and suicide attempts among transgender adults. *JAMA Psychiatry*, 77(1), 68–76.

Vigna, A. J., Poehlmann-Tynan, J., & Koenig, B. W. (2018). Does self-compassion facilitate resilience to stigma? A school-based study of sexual and gender minority youth. *Mindfulness*, 9(3), 914–924.

Vigna, A. J., Poehlmann-Tynan, J., & Koenig, B. W. (2020). Is self-compassion protective among sexual-and gender-minority adolescents across racial groups? *Mindfulness, 11*, 1–16.

Young, L. E., Jonas, A. B., Michaels, S., Jackson, J. D., Pierce, M. L., Schneider, J. A., & uConnect Study Team. (2017). Social-structural properties and HIV prevention among young men who have sex with men in the ballroom house and independent gay family communities. *Social Science & Medicine, 174*, 26–34.

8

COMPLEX TRAUMA AND POST-TRAUMATIC STRESS AMONG SGM CLIENTS

Introduction

Sexual and gender minority (SGM) individuals are exposed to a number of stressors in their lives that may lead to the development of traumatic responses. This is somewhat unsurprising, given the degree of anti-SGM animus that is so pervasive in global news and political discourse around the globe. Disparate treatment begins early in life. Within the home, disparities begin early as SGM individuals report experiencing greater levels of intrafamilial abuse, even in comparison to siblings (Balsam et al., 2005). Bullying within schools also disparately impacts SGM people, may begin early in school, and may lead to post-traumatic stress disorder (PTSD; Beckerman & Auerbach, 2014). Some elements of the minority stress model have been found to intersect with the development of trauma symptoms, such as internalized homonegativity among sexual minority people who have experienced sexual trauma (Solomon et al., 2019). There is also an intersection between gender role norms, heterosexism, and the experience of trauma that has been observed in the experiences of sexual minority individuals (Oringher & Samuelson, 2011; Szymanski & Balsam, 2011). Gender minority people are exposed to a number of types of trauma, ranging from interpersonal violence to collective trauma, that may lead to both PTSD and complex PTSD (e.g., Richmond et al., 2012). Environmental risk factors related to substance use and gender minority stress may also lead to a greater susceptibility to a trauma reaction among gender minority individuals (McCann & Brown, 2018). As an expert in SGM trauma once noted, "As long as the majority of cultures and contexts define non-heterosexual desires as deviant, sinful, or illegal, LGBT people will experience normative traumata arising from the experiences of being alive and queer" (Brown, 2003).

Treating trauma

There are a number of evidence-based approaches available for the treatment of trauma, many incorporating some degree of exposure (Difede et al., 2014). A minority stress informed approach that acknowledges the variety of stressors in the environment that may exacerbate or complicate trauama treatment is helpful in working with SGM clients (e.g., Shipherd et al., 2019). There is some guidance describing interventions with SGM clients that can provide illustrative examples of types of trauma, the execution of various trauma therapies, and what this may look like with given SGM populations (e.g., Pantalone et al., 2017). Eye movement desensitization and reprocessing (EMDR), for example, has been described in practice with sexual minority clients (O'Brien, 2017). The specific challenge in developing a trauma treatment strategy for SGM clients, however, is that minority stress may serve as an additional and complicating source of distress that intersects with the presentation of trauma symptoms and complicates straightforward trauma narratives that a clinician may associate with discreet instances of trauma. In work with SGM veterans, a population exposed to minority stress, microaggressions, and high levels of traumatic events, it has been noted that treatment gaps exist in implementing treatment as usual that may be further exacerbated by institutional discrimination (Livingston et al., 2019).

Given the association between experiential avoidance and trauma (e.g., Gold et al., 2011), in my own clinical practice with SGM clients I have introduced a number of the strategies described in Chapters 3–5 intended to begin a basic exposure to unwanted emotions and the practice of willingness to experience them in the service of living a more meaningful life (e.g., Walser & Westrup, 2007). Though there is some support for ACT as a standalone intervention for PTSD and this may be sufficient for some clients, I have found that needs vary (e.g., Wharton et al., 2019). For some clients with severe trauma symptoms and major traumatic experiences this serves as a precursor to prolonged exposure (Foa et al., 2007). In this way, there has also been an opportunity for a trusting relationship to have been built, and the preliminary experience with emotional exposure intrinsic in ACT facilitates acceptance of prolonged exposure.

Racial trauma

In recent years, specific clinical attention has turned to the trauma response that occurs due to pervasive racism, particularly anti-Black racism, in the United States (Helms, Nicolas, & Green, 2010). As noted in Chapter 4, the Black community is regularly subjected to images of the bodies of Black individuals who have died, including viral footage of deaths in which Black individuals are depicted in the process of being killed (Aymer, 2016). These profound stressors, in addition to frequent experiences of microaggressions, lead to PTSD symptoms even in the absence of a personal experience that meets criterion 1A for a traditional diagnosis (e.g., Williams et al., 2018). This phenomena increases the importance of SGM competent therapists to also be familiar with the experiences that SGM people of color may bring to treatment. For SGM people of color, while either identity may be a source of traumatic experience, the context of each individual determines which source of bias is more salient in each individual's life (e.g., Hughes & Hurtado, 2018).

Protocols for treating the effects of racial trauma are actively being developed in light of these findings within the realm of trauma-informed psychotherapy (e.g., Chavez-Dueñas et al., 2019; Comas-Díaz, 2016; Tummala-Narra, 2005), as well as tools to aid in clinical assessment (Williams et al., 2018). These protocols carry certain common threads, such as openly considering the full impact that racism has had on one's self, exploring and processing how this affects the self and behaviors moving through the world, and ultimately considering how this awareness changes one's behavior in the world. Many models conceptualize the final step as activism, as deeply opening one's self to the harms of racism and recognizing how its pervasiveness has shaped one's own world may inspire a desire to create change in the world. More recent adaptations include exploration of psychedelic-assisted psychotherapy for racial trauma (Williams et al., 2020). Though findings are not yet published, a study clinician and self-identified sexual minority person of color who is a treatment therapist for the ongoing trial experienced MDMA as a part of the therapist training protocol (Ching, 2020). He found the experience particularly helpful in exploring disonnance between his intersectional identities, and describes how the experience facilitated a greater sense of internal harmony. Additional research is needed into the needs of SGM people of color experiencing racial trauma, and an SGM competent clinician should continue to monitor this growing literature.

Complex trauma

Complex trauma refers to a trauamtic stressor that occurs repeatedly and cumulatively, and may provide a particularly important lens into the experiences of SGM people who report chronic traumatic events (e.g., Courtois, 2004). Though the specific meaning of complex trauma has varied over decades of research, examples have included ongoing childhood abuse, domestic violence, acute medical emergencies, or other adverse childhood events – particularly those in which the perpetrator was an attachment figure. Complex trauma symptoms include those generally attributed to PTSD, though include challenges with interpersonal relationships and trust as well as specific challenges in meaning-making (Courtois, 2004). Based upon the assumption that previously warm childhood relationships may have ended in rejection or rupture, some researchers have specifically recruited gender minority individuals in order to develop assessment measures of complex trauma (Maggiora Vergano et al., 2015). This instrument has been successfully used subsequently in exploring the relationship between complex trauma and well-being in a gender minority sample (Giovanardi et al., 2018), though it is still too lengthy for routine clinical use.

The sequenced, relationship-based approach to treating complex trauma has been developed as an extension of research into the unique elements of complex trauma (Courtois & Ford, 2012). The emphasis in this approach, based on research into the experience of complex trauma, is to strategically progress through treating those behaviors likely to be most disruptive in the individual's life, including interpersonal patterns that may interfere with the therapeutic relationship. Though there are no published examples of the application of the sequenced, relationship-based approach with SGM clients, in many ways the process follows the relative order of therapeutic processes outlined in this volume. First, it notes strategies that may reduce avoidance behaviors, as covered in Chapter 4. As avoidance of stressors is reduced, the emphasis shifts to the therapeutic relationship. As noted, a hallmark of complex trauma is the likely precursor of the betrayal of trust by a meaningful other, as well as ongoing disruption within interpersonal relationships. The relationship-building strategies described in Chapter 6 are a helpful guide for deepening the therapeutic relationship as a place where trust can be experienced.

Case example

Charles is a 44-year-old, cisgender, Black gay man living with HIV who entered therapy for anger management. During the course of the intake he disclosed that the current concern began at work. He was startled as he ended his day to find that police officers were waiting outside, and learned that a White person had called the police following a brief exchange of tense words when he was cut off entering the parking lot after their lunch break. He was initially overwhelmed by what the repercussions might be, as he is tall with a large frame and had past experiences of this evoking nervousness with White strangers. The police officers wrote a citation, which occurred just outside of his place of work, and Charles felt both degraded by the experience and angry that none of his co-workers of many years stopped to see if he was okay. He considered himself lucky to have had no major interactions with police prior to this, as most of his friends had stories that were more uncomfortable than his own. In initial interactions he was reserved and uncomfortable in the process of setting an appointment and providing referral information.

The first session would begin similar to this:

Therapist: I wonder if you can tell me a little more about why you're here?

Charles: You've seen the form. I need 15 sessions of anger management. Is there some sort of plan you follow we can just get out of the way?

T: Sure, there's a general range of topics we could cover under that. I wonder if you could tell me a little bit more about this situation? When I look at your slip from the court, this situation seems quite minor to lead to this kind of referral. I'm also aware that I'm sitting here as a White man noting this, though you're a quite tall Black man, and I imagine that leads other people to have certain responses to you?

C: You don't have to tell me. I walk into a door and get looks from people like I've just shouted a threat.

T: I know we're both aware of what has been in the news lately, as well, with police responses to Black men. I imagine there are many things that you do feel anger about, and also life has told you like in your situation that you can be seen as angry just existing.

C: It is one thing after another. What are you going to tell me, to express my anger? Because that sounds like terrible advice.

T: No, I know I don't understand this like you do. I wonder if I can help in exploring ways to feel what you haven't been able to feel yet. I noticed in the intake paperwork that you're also gay, which may have led you to my practice, and living with HIV. How does this all intersect?

C: I wanted to find a therapist at an LGBT clinic. Which means crossing town to get here. Though tying it with HIV reminds me of when I first got sick. All the places to test or be seen were either on the north side where the White gays lived, or downtown.

T: Okay … so it does sound like things have added up for a long time. What else can you tell me about this most recent experience?

C: You know … I've had nightmares about the situation going down differently. So many videos go around of men like me getting shot, getting choked. I shouted "nice turn signal" out of my window and this happened.

T: So you're experiencing nightmares. What else have you noticed?

This may be one way that therapy begins. There are a number of factors here to consider specifically relevant to SGM psychotherapy. First, there is a long history of LGBT or HIV centers being displaced from where communities of color live in many cities in the United States. This poses certain challenges to receiving care, as proximity is a strong indicator of attending an LGBT center for services, and more SGM individuals indicate an interest in care at an SGM community center than report having received such services (e.g., Martos et al., 2019). Note also that the clinician introduces the topic of race. As a supervisor, I have noted that often those possessing majority identities defer to a client to raise the topic if it concerns them. This seems more likely, in my experience, to give the client the indirect message that racial differences (or gender differences, etc.) cannot be discussed. For this reason, I have advised trainees to raise the issue first and remove the cultural taboo against discussing identity differences that exist in this culture. Also, note that his experiences relate to the intersection of his identities, as he both seeks opportunities to engage in the SGM community and notes that in his particular city, much of it is built up in a different part of the city than he lives.

This case also relates back to the descriptions above of complex trauma and the possibility of racial trauma. Charles describes having nightmares related to his recent experience that connect with current events regarding an awareness of police violence toward the Black community. There are also unexplored challenges related to his seroconversion and his coming out, as minority stress factors are considered. Urban areas in the United States vary significantly in terms of the level of racial integration in the gay community, and whether or not there are specific spaces for sexual minority men of color to meet. Finally, he has described how his stature and the color of his skin affect others' perception of his emotions, and indicates that he has adopted a habit of overcontrol. I would be concerned that if he has generally successfully overcontrolled revealing anger, he may more broadly mute his expressions of emotions or experience anxiety when expressing other types of affect.

Similar to the sequenced, relationship-based approach, we would begin therapy exploring avoidance behaviors. In this case, it may be the general expression of emotion, and we could begin with risk-taking around whatever emotions Charles identifies that he would like to express more. As this occurs in tandem with allowing himself to feel and express emotions within therapy, I would incorporate in the relational processes described in Chapter 6, so that we might built a trusting, warm relationship in session. At this point we might proceed with exploring his history and trauma responses that may benefit from a more formal, exposure-based approach. It would also be important to consider consent at each stage. A client like Charles may be open to a longer therapy to explore these concerns, or he may prefer to consider a brief plan that fits within his 15 required sessions. This should be considered and openly discussed at the first session, as well as how it would incorporate themes required by the court, if any exist. In my own practice, I am most comfortable using prolonged exposure when a client is open to an exposure-based therapy, though there are other evidence-based models available. Mapping the role of racial and complex trauma on the SORC appears on Table 8.1.

This SORC remains incomplete, as his provider would hope to learn more about Charles's methods of coping as well as how others outside of

Table 8.1 SORC of the Function of Racial and Complex Trauma

Stimulus	Organism	Response	Consequence
Charles is a tall Black man.	Charles described nightmares and should be assessed for other intrusive thoughts.	Charles may restrict emotional disclosures.	Coworkers may respond to Charles as if he were intimidating.
Charles is living with HIV.		Charles may limit social interactions with his colleagues.	The provider may experience Charles as guarded.
Charles identifies as gay, and prefers clinicians who are a part of the SGM community.	Charles has experienced structural barriers and challenges to accessing care in the past.		
The police were called on Charles recently, and he has been court ordered to attend anger management courses.	Charles has fears about interactions with police.		
Charles is overexposed to media images of police violence toward Black men.	"I cannot trust my co-workers to be concerned with my safety."		

work respond to him. He may appear warm or open with the provider in a way that differs from his presentation at work, where a recent inter-personal betrayal has occurred. There is also a possibility of an increase in intrusive thoughts or panic related to another police call that are elicited when he is leaving work or in the parking lot. With an awareness of the relationship between stress, distractibility, and medication adherence, his provider should also check in regarding his current adherence with his anti-retroviral medications.

Conclusion

SGM individuals are exposed to a variety of traumas, including dis-criminatory actions or violence beginning in childhood, assault in adult-hood, complex trauma related to the loss of family and parental rejection, or racial trauma that may or may not intersect with an SGM identity. It is important for a skilled provider to consider how minority stress intersects with or is exacerbated by other sources of trauma in the client's life, as well as if preliminary psychotherapy should occur before initiating an exposure-based therapy.

Key points

- SGM people are susceptible to a variety of traumas across the lifespan.
- Parental abuse or rejection may contribute to the development of complex trauma, which is characterized by a loss in interpersonal trust and a sense of meaning.
- Racial trauma among SGM people of color may or may not intersect with their other identities, though this should be explored by the therapist.

Recommended reading

Alvarez, A. N., Liang, C. T. H., & Neville, H. A. (2016). *The cost of racism for people of color: Contextualizing experiences of discrimination*. American Psychological Association.

Eckstrand, K. L., & Potter, J. (Eds.). (2017). *Trauma, resilience, and health promotion in LGBT patients: What every healthcare provider should know*. Springer.

Nadal, K. (2018). *Microaggressions and trauamtic stress: Theory, research, and clinical treatment.* American Psychological Association.

Walser, R., & Westrup, D. (2007). *Acceptance and commitment therapy for the treatment of post-traumatic stress disorder and trauma-related problems: A practitioner's guide to using mindfulness and acceptance strategies.* New Harbinger Publications.

References

Alvarez, A. N., Liang, C. T. H. & Neville, H. A. (2016). *Cultural, racial, and ethnic psychology book series. The cost of racism for people of color: Contextualizing experiences of discrimination.* Washington, D.C.: American Psychological Association.

Aymer, S. R. (2016). 'I can't breathe': A case study-helping Black men cope with race-related trauma stemming from police killing and brutality. *Journal of Human Behavior in the Social Environment, 26,* 367–376.

Beckerman, N. L., & Auerbach, C. (2014). PTSD as aftermath for bullied LGBT adolescents: The case for comprehensive assessment. *Social Work in Mental Health, 12*(3), 195–211.

Balsam, K. F., Rothblum, E. D., & Beauchaine, T. P. (2005). Victimization over the life span: A comparison of lesbian, gay, bisexual, and heterosexual siblings. *Journal of Consulting and Clinical Psychology, 73,* 477–487.

Brown, L.S. (2003). Sexuality, lies, and loss: Lesbian, gay, and bisexual perspectives on trauma. *Journal of Trauma Practice, 2,* 55–68.

Chavez-Dueñas, N. Y., Adames, H. Y., Perez-Chavez, J. G., & Salas, S. P. (2019). Healing ethno-racial trauma in Latinx immigrant communities: Cultivating hope, resistance, and action. *American Psychologist, 74*(1), 49–62.

Ching, T. H. (2020). Intersectional insights from an MDMA-assisted psychotherapy training trial: An open letter to racial/ethnic and sexual/gender minorities. *Journal of Psychedelic Studies, 4*(1), 61–68.

Comas-Díaz, L. (2016). Racial trauma recovery: A race-informed therapeutic approach to racial wounds. In A. N. Alvarez, C. T. H. Liang, & H. A. Neville (Eds.), *Cultural, racial, and ethnic psychology book series. The cost of racism for people of color: Contextualizing experiences of discrimination* (pp. 249–272). Washington, D.C.: American Psychological Association.

Courtois, C. A. (2004). Complex trauma, complex reactions: Assessment and treatment. *Psychotherapy: Theory, Research, & Practice, 41,* 412–425.

Courtois, C. A., & Ford, J. D. (2012). *Treatment of complex trauma: A sequenced, relationship-based approach.* New York, NY: Guilford Press.

Difede, J., Olden, M., & Cukor, J. (2014). Evidence-based treatment of post-traumatic stress disorder. *Annual Review of Medicine, 65,* 319–332.

Eckstrand, K. L., & Potter, J. (Eds.). (2017). *Trauma, resilience, and health promotion in LGBT patients: What every healthcare provider should know.* New York, NY: Springer.

Foa, E., Hembree, E., & Rothbaum, B. O. (2007). *Prolonged exposure therapy for PTSD: Emotional processing of traumatic experiences therapist guide.* New York, NY: Oxford University Press.

Giovanardi, G., Vitelli, R., Maggiora Vergano, C., Fortunato, A., Chianura, L., Lingiardi, V., & Speranza, A. M. (2018). Attachment patterns and complex trauma in a sample of adults diagnosed with gender dysphoria. *Frontiers in Psychology, 9*(60), 1–13.

Gold, S. D., Feinstein, B. A., Skidmore, W. C., & Marx, B. P. (2011). Childhood physical abuse, internalized homophobia, and experiential avoidance among lesbians and gay men. *Psychological Trauma: Theory, Research, Practice, and Policy, 3*(1), 50–60.

Helms, J. E., Nicolas, G., & Green, C. E. (2010). Racism and ethnoviolence as trauma: Enhancing professional training. *Traumatology, 16,* 53–62.

Hughes, B. E., & Hurtado, S. (2018). Thinking about sexual orientation: College experiences that predict identity salience. *Journal of College Student Development, 59,* 309–326.

Livingston, N. A., Berke, D. S., Ruben, M. A., Matza, A. R., & Shipherd, J. C. (2019). Experiences of trauma, discrimination, microaggressions, and minority stress among trauma-exposed LGBT veterans: Unexpected findings and unresolved service gaps. *Psychological Trauma: Theory, Research, Practice, and Policy, 11*(7), 695–703.

Maggiora Vergano, C., Lauriola, M., & Speranza, A. M. (2015). The complex trauma questionnaire (ComplexTQ): Development and preliminary psychometric properties of an instrument for measuring early relational trauma. *Frontiers in Psychology, 6*(1323), 1–13.

Martos, A. J., Fingerhut, A., Wilson, P. A., & Meyer, I. H. (2019). Utilization of LGBT-specific clinics and providers across three cohorts of lesbian, gay, and bisexual people in the United States. *SSM-Population Health, 9,* 100505.

McCann, E., & Brown, M. (2018). Vulnerability and psychosocial risk factors regarding people who Identify as transgender. A systematic review of the research evidence. *Issues in Mental Health Nursing, 39*(1), 3–15.

Nadal, K. (2018). *Microaggressions and trauamtic stress: Theory, research, and clinical treatment.* Washington, D.C.: American Psychological Association.

O'Brien, J. M. (2017). EMDR therapy with lesbian/gay/bisexual clients. In M. Nickerson (Ed.), *Cultural competence and healing culturally based trauma with EMDR therapy: Innovative strategies and protocols* (pp. 195–208). New York, NY: Springer.

Oringher, J., & Samuelson, K. W. (2011). Intimate partner violence and the role of masculinity in male same-sex relationships. *Traumatology, 17*(2), 68–74.

Pantalone, D. W., Valentine, S. E., & Shipherd, J. C. (2017). Working with survivors of trauma in the sexual minority and transgender and gender nonconforming populations. In K. A. DeBord, A. R. Fischer, K. J. Bieschke, & R. M. Perez (Eds.), *Handbook of sexual orientation and gender diversity in counseling and psychotherapy* (pp. 183–211). Washington, D.C.: American Psychological Association.

Richmond, K. A., Burnes, T., & Carroll, K. (2012). Lost in trans-lation: Interpreting systems of trauma for transgender clients. *Traumatology, 18*(1), 45–57.

Shipherd, J. C., Berke, D., & Livingston, N. A. (2019). Trauma recovery in the transgender and gender diverse community: Extensions of the minority stress model for treatment planning. *Cognitive and Behavioral Practice, 26*(4), 629–646.

Solomon, D. T., Combs, E. M., Allen, K., Roles, S., DiCarlo, S., Reed, O., & Klaver, S. J. (2019). The impact of minority stress and gender identity on PTSD outcomes in sexual minority survivors of interpersonal trauma. *Psychology & Sexuality.* Advance article online. https://doi.org/10.1080/19419899.2019.1690033.

Szymanski, D. M., & Balsam, K. F. (2011). Insidious trauma: Examining the relationship between heterosexism and lesbians' PTSD symptoms. *Traumatology, 17*(2), 4–13.

Tummala-Narra, P. (2005). Addressing political and racial terror in the therapeutic relationship. *American Journal of Orthopsychiatry, 75*(1), 19–26.

Walser, R., & Westrup, D. (2007). *Acceptance and commitment therapy for the treatment of post-traumatic stress disorder and trauma-related problems: A practitioner's guide to using mindfulness and acceptance strategies.* New Harbinger Publications.

Wharton, E., Edwards, K. S., Juhasz, K., & Walser, R. D. (2019). Acceptance-based interventions in the treatment of PTSD: Group and individual pilot data using Acceptance and Commitment Therapy. *Journal of Contextual Behavioral Science, 14,* 55–64.

Williams, M. T., Metzger, I. W., Leins, C., & DeLapp, C. (2018). Assessing racial trauma within a DSM–5 framework: The UConn racial/ethnic stress & trauma survey. *Practice Innovations, 3*(4), 242–260.

Williams, M. T., Reed, S., & Aggarwal, R. (2020). Culturally informed research design issues in a study for MDMA-assisted psychotherapy for posttraumatic stress disorder. *Journal of Psychedelic Studies, 4*(1), 40–50.

9

HEALTH CONSIDERATIONS AMONG SGM CLIENTS

Introduction

Minority stress does not only affect psychological well-being, it has also been associated with health disparites (e.g., Williams & Mann, 2017). As noted previously, the powerful impact of HIV on both sexual and gender minority (SGM) communities, as well as its role as a driver of SGM behavioral research, means that particularly when considering sexual minority men and trans women, a great deal is known about psychological factors that relate to sexual behavior, substance use, and the association of these factors with risk-taking, condomless sex, and general psychological well-being. Few populations have been as heavily researched in terms of medical trust and mistrust, medication adherence, or behavior change in response to information than SGM people. The unfortunate converse of this is also true – less is known about health behaviors and populations less associated with HIV. This is despite evidence of a variety of physical health complaints that occur more frequently in the presence of minority stress –

particularly prejudicial events (e.g., Frost, Lehavot, & Meyer 2015). Such reported disparities range from a poor general assessment of one's health to increases in rates of cancer diagnoses, cardiovascular risks, and diabetes (e.g., Lick et al., 2013).

Medical settings are also rife with microaggressions, mistreatment, and cultural insensitivity. Femme lesbians are encouraged to consider birth control despite no reported sex with men, queer men are lectured about sexual behaviors with little nuance and with insulting language, and trans and non-binary patients are routinely misgendered, from check-in through post-visit charting. Commonly reported barriers for gender minority in-dividuals range from lack of access and providers who are not culturally competent to prejudicial encounters while receiving treatment (Safer et al., 2016). Among sexual minority women, those who identify as butch report greater mistreatment, fewer gynecological exams, and greater difficulty identifying culturally competent health care (Hiestand et al., 2007). This chapter will only touch on some of the common areas in which health considerations may be important for your SGM clients.

Clinical health psychology 101

It helps to begin to consider the standards and norms of the discipline of clinical health psychology. My bias in approaching the content in this chapter is that I completed a postdoctoral fellowship in HIV behavioral medicine after I received my degree, and became board certified in clinical health psychology in 2012. I note this because while such training is not required in most healthcare systems, it exposed me to the norms of clinical health psychology that are not often considered in other parts of the field. For example, the onset of hormone replacement therapy (HRT) may lead to a number of changes in the experience and expression of one's mood, and while this is a relatively normative experience, psychologists who work in this area should be aware of and monitor their client's experience in case adjustments are needed by their medical provider. Individuals newly diagnosed with HIV may struggle to mentally prepare for a daily medical regimen, or fear stigma that they believe may affect them. Despite changes in medication regimens and increased awareness of their effec-tiveness, initiating antiretroviral therapy is still generally experienced as a life-changing action (Bruton et al., 2018). Finally, one of the largest recent changes in SGM practice has been the role of pre-exposure prophylactic (PrEP) medications to reduce the likelihood of seroconversion, though there are still barriers to access and adoption based on race, ethnicity, and whether or not someone lives in an urban area within the United States (Brooks et al., 2019; Hubach et al., 2017; Young et al., 2018). The ways in which SGM individuals' lives encounter medical systems and incorporate pharmaceutical agents differ from what a therapist who primarily works with the general population may expect.

HIV and PrEP

HIV has had profound effects on SGM communities, and still holds a central place in the politics and social organization of sexual minority men's lives. In a relatively short period of time, however, this has led to stark generational divides within the community (Hammack et al., 2019). A gay man who came out in the early 1980s may belong to a generation that experienced a great deal of death and the first wave of the HIV pandemic, may be a long-term survivor living with HIV, and has never known a gay community without HIV (Halkitis, 2013). A gay man who came out in the 2010s is aware of HIV, though he may be taking PrEP and consider his personal life and sexual choices to be less centered around HIV prevention. Some of his SGM friends are married, and in urban areas he is less likely to have considered whether or not being out would affect his career prospects. If he has been diagnosed with HIV, he is likely aware that his life span will be comparable to a seronegative person if he is adherent to his medications (e.g., May et al., 2012), though younger men of color still face disproportionate risks of seroconverting (e.g., Parker et al., 2017).

In my own work exploring the experiences of sexual minority men living with HIV, reports of internalized stigma related to the diagnosis and concern regarding stigma from others are still high among some men (Skinta et al., 2014; 2015). This was true despite my past work occurring in San Francisco, which has both a large gay community as well as a large number of HIV-oriented service organizations and social groups. Some sources of stigma described came from family members, still fearful of contracting HIV through casual contact, whereas others were attributed to negative experiences prior to the availability of PrEP, when potential partners harshly rejected these men upon learning of their serostatus. In more recent work I have done (Skinta et al., 2020), there do appear to be shifts in the experience of men in urban areas where PrEP adoption has become widespread. In my private practice, I have found that asking SGM clients about their use or knowledge of PrEP to be helpful in guiding discussions around how they care for their bodies and the thoughts or fears they express related to HIV, PrEP side effects, or both.

Writing a pretreatment letter

The requirements of a letter prior to gender-affirming medical procedures has a complicated and controversial history, primarily due to the gate-keeping role this allowed providers to take during the assessment (Lev, 2006). When the process first became standardized, neither the gender minority stress model nor gender-affirming models of care had been developed (Keo-Meier & Fitzgerald, 2017). This led to a variety of challenges for gender minority people seeking affirmative care, and there is a large body of literature describing the role of the therapist as a "gate-keeper" in a manner that is no longer considered appropriate. A presurgical psychological evaluation should include information that most psychologists are skilled at gathering in the course of a standard intake, information that may be necessary for a medical provider to be aware of possible complications that could occur in post-surgical follow-up, as well as the opportunity for the assessor to identify any supportive actions that may need to occur prior to surgery (Block & Marek, 2019). Following a mental status exam to determine that an individual is capable of understanding the risks and benefits of the procedure, a letter should focus on relevant history, particularly health behaviors (e.g., adherence with past medications, awareness of any behavior changes required during recuperation or to facilitate healing, appointment attendance, trust in their medical provider). Some concerns are particularly relevant, as, like most surgeries, gender-affirming surgeries heal more slowly and the likelihood of complications increase if the individual is a current smoker (Feldman, 2008). A good letter should speak to follow-up care, and should use the current name and pronouns used by the client to the greatest extent possible. If the insurer or surgeon requires the letter to include a legal name that differs and is on an insurance policy, then with consent of the patient that should be included as a parenthetical. The clinician writing the letter should be familiar with any legal requirements in their state that may necessitate variations of these recommendations. While the letter should be specific to the procedure being requested (not a generic letter for "gender-affirming procedures"), in my experience there is considerable latitude depending on the context and the recipient. For example, I have worked with some endocrinologists and surgeons in situations where the client's insurance plan only requires a form to approve payment from the medical provider, and they certify that they have received pre-intervention letters. In those cases, the offices are able to receive letters that make no superfluous reference to a former name or gender pronoun, as the client has already established care and their medical provider has their own internal system of record keeping inclusive of the client's current name.

In most cases, an official diagnosis of gender dysphoria must be included to meet requirements for both third-party payers and the medical provider. This is the case despite the seventh edition of the *WPATH Standards of Care* noting that not all gender minority individuals experience dysphoria (World Professional Association for Transgender Health, 2012). This diagnosis has a complex history, and gender minority clients have different relationships with it. I have had clients who celebrate having the diagnosis applied as a roadblock to be cleared to pursue the life they wish to lead, as well as those who find it offensive and a necessary evil in order to receive services. It may be helpful as early in the assessment process as possible to discuss this with your client, and if it is required for documentation related to services that the client is pursuing, to dedicate space and time if the client would like to process their reaction first. In this way, an affirming process to letter writing might still center on client autonomy while meeting any legal and ethical standards of practice.

Finally, there is a role of advocacy and familiarity with your local community in order to effectively assist clients who are seeking gender-affirming procedures. Clients who are uncertain where to begin their journey in their insurance plan may be exposed to microaggressions prior to discovering an affirming provider in their network. Further, 20% of gender minority individuals report a non-binary or genderqueer identity (Richards et al., 2016), some of whom seek gender-affirming surgical interventions without a binary gender as the destination. Such desired interventions may include microdoses of HRT that result in more modest feminization or masculinization of the body, masculinizing chest surgeries, and a variety of genital surgeries. Though access has increased, some non-binary procedures, such as penectomy/ orchiectomy without vulvoplasty, are still only offered by a small number of providers within the United States (e.g., Richards et al., 2017). Affirmative care includes being aware of what service providers offer services in your area, and how best to aid your client in navigating those services.

Case example

Xan is a 23-year-old non-binary Asian-American who has requested a letter for top surgery (bilateral mastectomy with free nipple graft). Xan came out to their parents when they were 15, and with their parent's support legally changed their name to a less gendered alternative at age 18. They consulted with an endocrinologist when they were 19 regarding the possibility of receiving microdoses of testosterone, though upon further self-exploration and research decided that this was not an option they wanted to pursue at that time. When they asked their provider to write a letter, the provider reviewed both Xan's intake and regular self-assessment forms in the clinic, and prepared a session to review the risks and recovery plan that Xan's doctor had faxed to her office. As described previously, the provider conferred with Xan about the need to include a diagnosis of gender dys-phoria in the letter, which Xan approved. The therapist completed the letter following that session, and reviewed it with Xan prior to sending it to the surgeon's office the following week. Though alternate scheduling would have been possible if there were time factors, in this case Xan preferred the option to review the letter first with their provider, as the dates the surgeon had available to schedule left ample advance time. The letter looked like this:

Dear Dr. Eric Green,

I am the psychologist working with your patient, Mx. Xan Mauve (DOB: 09/22/1996). Xan is a 23-year-old, non-binary (assigned female at birth), Asian-American individual who has requested an assessment to receive a bilateral mastectomy with free nipple graft. They began receiving services in my private practice in September, 2019, and prior to this assessment had received 15, 50-minute sessions with me. During this time I have gotten to know Mx. Mauve, and can speak to their history. Xan described growing up in a progressive suburb without many gender divisions, so did not begin to experience a sense of difference until middle school when their peers began to divide by gender to engage in different activities. They described a process of self-exploration, reading online, and asking questions of trusted adults about gender identity. By 15 years old, Xan felt confident that they identified as non-binary and came out to their parents. Their parents have been consistently supportive since that time, and aided Xan in the process of pursuing a legal name change at the age of 18.

Xan meets appropriate criteria for F64.1 Gender Dysphoria. Xan carries no additional diagnoses at this time, and is receiving psychological services oriented toward general self-exploration and life planning. Per their history, their only major medical event was a broken arm while skateboarding at age 12, and this healed without incident. Xan's mother is a medical doctor, so Xan has a positive view of medical professionals and feels that all of their questions about the procedure, risks, and benefits have been described in their sessions with you. They reported experimenting with nicotine products their freshman year of college, where they smoked 1–2 cigarettes at parties for approximately six months. At that time, Xan had a conversation with an older trans friend who informed them about the risks this could lead to if they ever pursued top surgery. At that point Xan quit and reported no nicotine intake since. They reported no other substance use, only occasional alcohol consumption, such as champagne on the New Year.

Xan is eager to proceed with their surgery. They have used a binder to flatten their breasts since approximately 18 years old, though recently with occasional discomfort. They exercise regularly, and most discomfort associated with binding occurs during exercise. They described post-surgical care and the timeline to resume athletic activities that were provided by your office.

Though you will make the final medical determination, I have found no reason that psychological factors would interfere with proceeding at this time. Please feel free to contact my office as needed, at 773-555-5555.

Sue D'aunym, Psy.D., ABPP
Board-Certified Health Psychologist
License #PSY2JX99

As you may note in this letter, the flow is relatively brief, and is focused on the needs of the client. As a diagnosis was required, gender dysphoria is noted. The letter covers the client's medical history, factors likely to affect compliance with medical care, substance use, and the client's awareness and ability to recite back important information regarding their plan with their provider. It is generally preferred when necessary to refer to an assigned or designated sex at birth, rather than alternatives that emphasize biological essentialism. Though a history of the client's gender identification is provided as support for the diagnosis, it is not done so in an overly invasive way and emphasizes details relevant to the referral. In this case, for instance, the exploration and decision not to pursue HRT was not included, though could be upon specific request. In my experience, gender-affirming medical providers are equally working from a place of client autonomy rather than gate-keeping, and will quickly follow up or request revisions if there is something incomplete for their purposes within a letter.

COVID-19 and SGM health

The spread of COVID-19 at the start of 2020 and subsequent global efforts to mitigate the pandemic such as shelter-in-place orders, travel restrictions, and the deferral of non-essential medical care affected SGM people in a variety of ways. Some of the impact was due directly to the social effect of confinement, though other changes highlight the ubiquity of anti-SGM bias that are still common around the world. The deferral of non-essential medical care postponed gender-affirming medical procedures and appointments in most countries and may have created obstacles to the initiation or monitoring of HIV-related health. Though the restrictions in place at the time this book is being written are assumed to be finite, important lessons might be drawn from current events.

Bias and discriminatory actions toward SGM people during the pandemic have generally taken two forms. The first is in the direct or indirect expression of hostility toward SGM people as some political and religious leaders blamed the community for the pandemic. Evangelical religious figures across the globe and in most faith traditions took the opportunity to describe the virus as a punishment for greater societal acceptance of SGM people (e.g., O'Connor, 2020). Another common form of discrimination or bias was the implementation of rules intended to prevent the spread of COVID-19 as justification to harass SGM people. A shelter in Uganda that provided services specifically for SGM people was raided and the residents arrested, ostensibly for hosting a crowd that might spread COVID-19

(Ghoshal, 2020). Some nations, including Panama, Ecuador, and Peru, initially made efforts to reduce citizens leaving their homes under shelter-in-place orders by designating a gender for each day (Perez-Brumer & Silva-Santisteban, 2020). That is, only women could run essential errands or shop on one day, only men on the next. Such rules quickly led to increased reports of police harassment of trans women, and such rules were eventually revoked.

Conclusion

Health disparities that affect SGM individuals occur due to a variety of reasons, with some adverse experiences mediated by minority stress processes. Informed clinicians should be aware of SGM stress and its impact on health and behavior, as well as medical needs that may be more commonly experienced within SGM communities. Heterocentric and ciscentric assumptions may create challenges for SGM individuals seeking healthcare services, and as the COVID pandemic has unfolded, unexpected events may lead to sudden changes in the experience of bias and subsequent health vulnerability. Though only a cursory introduction, therapists should seek out and be aware of health concerns that affect those populations that they work with.

Key points

- SGM health disparities extend to physical health, both generally as a result of exposure to environmental stressors, and through difficulty accessing specialty care.
- HIV remains a major touchstone in the lives of sexual minority men, resulting in major differences in generational experiences and views. This is particularly salient following the widespread availability of PrEP.
- Gender-affirming care is imperative for meeting the needs of gender minority people.

Recommended reading

Halkitis, P. N. (2013). *The AIDS generation: Stories of survival and resilience.* Oxford University Press.

Meyer, I. H., & Northridge, M. E. (2010). *The health of sexual minorities: Public* health perspectives on lesbian, gay, bisexual, and transgender populations. Springer.

World Professional Association for Transgender Health. (2012). *Standards of care for the health of transsexual, transgender, and gender-nonconforming people*. World Professional Association for Transgender Health.

References

Block, A. R., & Marek, R. J. (2019). Presurgical psychological evaluation: Risk factor identification and mitigation. *Journal of Clinical Psychology in Medical Settings, 27*, 396–405.

Brooks, R. A., Nieto, O., Landrian, A., & Donohoe, T. J. (2019). Persistent stigmatizing and negative perceptions of pre-exposure prophylaxis (PrEP) users: Implications for PrEP adoption among Latino men who have sex with men. *AIDS Care, 31*(4), 427–435.

Bruton, J., Rai, T., Day, S., & Ward, H. (2018). Patient perspectives on the HIV continuum of care in London: A qualitative study of people diagnosed between 1986 and 2014. *BMJ Open, 8*(3), e020208.

Feldman, J. (2008). Medical and surgical management of the transgender patient: What the primary care clinician. In H. J. Makadon, K. H. Mayer, J. Potter, & H. Goldhammer (Eds.). *The Fenway guide to lesbian, gay, bisexual, and transgender health* (pp. 365–392). Philadelphia, PA: American College of Physicians.

Frost, D. M., Lehavot, K., & Meyer, I. H. (2015). Minority stress and physical health among sexual minority individuals. *Journal of Behavioral Medicine, 38*(1), 1–8.

Ghoshal, N. (2020, April 3). Uganda LGBT shelter residents arrested on COVID-19 pretext. *Human Rights Watch: Dispatches.* https://www.hrw.org/news/2020/04/03/uganda-lgbt-shelter-residents-arrested-covid-19-pretext#.

Halkitis, P. N. (2013). *The AIDS generation: Stories of survival and resilience.* Oxford University Press.

Hammack, P. L., Toolis, E. E., Wilson, B. D., Clark, R. C., & Frost, D. M. (2019). Making meaning of the impact of pre-exposure prophylaxis (PrEP) on public health and sexual culture: Narratives of three generations of gay and bisexual men. *Archives of Sexual Behavior, 48*(4), 1041–1058.

Hiestand, K. R., Horne, S. G., & Levitt, H. M. (2007). Effects of gender identity on experiences of healthcare for sexual minority women. *Journal of LGBT Health Research, 3*(4), 15–27.

Hubach, R. D., Currin, J. M., Sanders, C. A., Durham, A. R., Kavanaugh, K. E., Wheeler, D. L., & Croff, J. M. (2017). Barriers to access and adoption of pre-exposure prophylaxis for the prevention of HIV among men who have sex with men (MSM) in a relatively rural state. *AIDS Education and Prevention, 29*(4), 315–329.

Keo-Meier, C. L., & Fitzgerald, K. M. (2017). Affirmative psychological testing and neurocognitive assessment with transgender adults. *Psychiatric Clinics, 40*(1), 51–64.

Lev, A. I. (2006). Disordering gender identity: Gender identity disorder in the DSM-IV-TR. *Journal of Psychology & Human Sexuality, 17*(3–4), 35–69.

Lick, D. J., Durso, L. E., & Johnson, K. L. (2013). Minority stress and physical health among sexual minorities. *Perspectives on Psychological Science, 8*(5), 521–548.

May, M., Gompels, M., & Sabin, C. (2012). Life expectancy of HIV-1-positive individuals approaches normal conditional on response to antiretroviral therapy: UK collaborative HIV cohort study. *Journal of the International AIDS Society, 15*, 18078.

Meyer, I. H., & Northridge, M. E. (2010). *The health of sexual minorities: Public health perspectives on lesbian, gay, bisexual, and transgender populations.* Springer.

O'Connor, R. (2020, April 2). DUP councillor blames gay marriage and abortion for coronavirus: 'You reap what you sow'. *The Irish Post.* https://www.irishpost.com/news/dup-councillor-blames-gay-marriage-abortion-coronavirus-reap-sow-182766.

Parker, C. M., Garcia, J., Philbin, M. M., Wilson, P. A., Parker, R. G., & Hirsch, J. S. (2017). Social risk, stigma and space: Key concepts for understanding HIV vulnerability among black men who have sex with men in New York City. *Culture, Health & Sexuality, 19*(3), 323–337.

Perez-Brumer, A., & Silva-Santisteban, A. (2020). COVID-19 policies can perpetuate violence against transgender communities: Insights from Peru. *AIDS & Behavior.* Advance article online. https://doi.org/10.1007/s10461-020-02889-z.

Richards, C., Bouman, W. P., & Barker, M. J. (Eds.). (2017). *Genderqueer and non-binary genders.* Springer.

Richards, C., Bouman, W. P., Seal, L., Barker, M. J., Nieder, T. O., & T'Sjoen, G. (2016). Non-binary or genderqueer genders. *International Review of Psychiatry, 28*(1), 95–102.

Safer, J. D., Coleman, E., Feldman, J., Garofalo, R., Hembree, W., Radix, A., & Sevelius, J. (2016). Barriers to health care for transgender individuals. *Current Opinion in Endocrinology, Diabetes, and Obesity, 23*(2), 168.

Skinta, M. D., Brandrett, B. D., & Margolis, E. (2020). Desiring intimacy and building community: young, gay and living with HIV in the time of PrEP. *Culture, Health & Sexuality*. Advance article online. https://doi.org/10.1080/13691058.2020.1795722.

Skinta, M. D., Brandrett, B. D., Schenk, W. C., Wells, G., & Dilley, J. W. (2014). Shame, self-acceptance and disclosure in the lives of gay men living with HIV: An interpretative phenomenological analysis approach. *Psychology & Health*, 29(5), 583–597.

Skinta, M. D., Lezama, M., Wells, G., & Dilley, J. W. (2015). Acceptance and compassion-based group therapy to reduce HIV stigma. *Cognitive and Behavioral Practice*, 22(4), 481–490.

Williams, S. L., & Mann, A. K. (2017). Sexual and gender minority health disparities as a social issue: How stigma and intergroup relations can explain and reduce health disparities. *Journal of Social Issues*, 73(3), 450–461.

World Professional Association for Transgender Health (2012). *Standards of care for the health of transsexual, transgender, and gender-nonconforming people*. World Professional Association for Transgender Health.

Young, L. E., Schumm, P., Alon, L., Bouris, A., Ferreira, M., Hill, B., ... Schneider, J. A. (2018). PrEP Chicago: A randomized controlled peer change agent intervention to promote the adoption of pre-exposure prophylaxis for HIV prevention among young Black men who have sex with men. *Clinical Trials*, 15(1), 44–52.

10

SPECIAL ETHICAL CONSIDERATIONS FOR SGM THERAPISTS

Introduction

Sexual and gender minority (SGM) therapists face a number of challenges when managing a clinical practice within the SGM community while simultaneously attempting to engage socially. This can be challenging on a number of levels. First and foremost, smartphone-based dating apps are one of the most common ways that sexual minority couples meet one another, at rates significantly higher than heterosexual couples (~70% vs. 20%; Rosenfeld & Thomas, 2012). This is primarily challenging given the lack of ethical guidance on the use of these apps, notwithstanding research suggestive of the role of this type of impersonal dating on the perpetuation of racism within communities of sexual minority men (Robinson, 2015). The rise of app-based dating, as well as traditional concerns related to the likelihood of multiple relationships within SGM communities, is the focus of this chapter. It should be noted that though the discussion presented here may be of interest to any provider considering ethical aspects of practice, I draw upon the Ethics Code of the American Psychological Association specifically in discussing boundaries and obligations (American Psychological Association, 2017).

Perspectives on multiple relationships and SGM psychotherapy

Though a review of the literature demonstrates periodic peaks in interest, there is not a density of literature specific to SGM identities that constitute the frequent exchange of perspectives present in many areas of the field. In an attempt to find an ethical discussion of one of the most popular apps used globally, as an example, I found only a footnote in an article on the ethics of dating for heterosexual couples that noted that apps specific to the gay community are only used for sex, so should never be used by therapists (e.g., Berlin, 2014). The challenge of finding community, or even romantic partners, is exacerbated through the high rate of closures of SGM venues over the past decade (Campkin & Marshall, 2017). As noted previously, however, Grindr is also the most frequent source of matches that lead to same-sex weddings. This is not a novel ethical question, however, as bars, dance clubs, and other community events have all been suggested to be inherently sexual in nature and potentially problematic (Gonsiorek, 1994; Lamb & Catanzaro, 1998). It should be of added concern that, to my knowledge, an ethical consideration of the potential for multiple relationships among gender minority therapists seeking gender minority supervisors or therapists for themselves has not yet been authored by a gender minority practitioner. Though some of the principles described in this chapter may be relevant, I will not conjecture specific recommendations for gender minority therapists in the absence of such a literature.

In practice, SGM therapists are members of small communities. This raises the likelihood that some contact not only may occur outside of therapy, but likely will occur if the therapist is an active member of the community or socializes in SGM-defined spaces (e.g., Graham & Liddle, 2009; Kessler & Waehler, 2005; Morrow, 2000). Some of the earliest publications to consider the ethical ramifications of SGM therapists encountering therapy clients in public emphasized the possibility of harm and encouraged minimizing contact (Brown, 1989; Lamb & Catanzaro, 1998). This seems problematic in other ways, however, as it is difficult to imagine an SGM therapist thriving and living an open and meaningful life without any community contact. Literature on sources of SGM resilience frequently recommend both community connection as well as active means of coping with political stressors such as engaging in activism (Russell & Richards, 2003). An ethical consideration of SGM therapist involvement in the community might consider the strong possibility of encounters outside of therapy, the potential posed by an overly strict interpretation of the Ethics Code that isolates the clinician, and the manner in which any contact might be compatible with the Ethics Code (e.g., Everett, MacFarlane, Reynolds, & Anderson, 2013).

Principle a: beneficence and non-maleficence

Principle A of the Ethics Code encourages the protection of rights and welfare of the communities, clients, and fellow professionals that we work with (American Psychological Association, 2017, Principle A). Bearing this in mind, community connection is a key resilience factor for SGM people (e.g., Pflum, Testa, Balsam, Goldblum, & Bongar, 2015), and loneliness a key driver of adverse outcomes in SGM communities (Mereish & Poteat, 2015). I would be concerned that both the rights and well-being of colleagues discouraged from involvement in the community, community spaces, or community culture would suffer. Relatedly, in ethical writings referring to another small community, deaf culture, it has been argued that clients should be entitled to accessing providers familiar with and active members of their community (e.g., Guthmann & Sandberg, 2002). Preventing such relationships would be deleterious to both the provider who trained as a therapist to work with and support their own community, as well as the client who seeks a therapy experience that does not require explanation of community norms, slang, or practices. I have heard multiple stories over the years of friends' experiences with therapists who frequently interrupt to ask for clarification on vocabulary or slang, or ask questions unrelated to the therapy to verify if rumors they have heard about the community are true or not. Refusing to treat individuals solely because of a potential dual relationship may deny a client the only culturally competent treatment available to them. While referring to another SGM provider if one believed the likelihood of contact is too high could potentially be possible in a dense, SGM neighborhood in a larger city, this assumption is still predicated upon factors of whether or not alternate providers are available, within network, or have the experience or therapeutic orientation sought by the client. This is more challenging in rural environments, where interdependence and familiarity already increase the possibility of multiple relationships (Campbell & Gordon, 2003; Schank & Skovholt, 1997).

This leads to a number of assumptions that are worth considering in diving deeper into the Ethics Code. First, as SGM spaces shrink even within larger cities, dating app use has become largely normative within SGM communities. Secondly, it has become possibly the most common way that many SGM people, particularly sexual minority men, meet romantic partners and eventual spouses. In rural communities, the possibility of multiple relationships is both high and potentially unavoidable for SGM community members. Finally, if an SGM therapist does use a dating app, there is a possibility that they will see clients on the apps, and that those clients will see them. This is not, however, an argument that multiple relationships are never avoidable or always harmless to clients. These assumptions suggest that the risk of multiple relationships remains pervasive, added to by the use of apps, and that a strict prohibition may be both difficult and potentially harmful to therapists who rely on community contact for resilience. What is needed is a considered middle ground.

Morrow (2000) suggests that SGM therapists have three options when it comes to the potential for multiple relationships. The first is to set and maintain strict boundaries that may ultimately harm the therapeutic relationship. An example may be to consider the effect of constantly leaving a bar, social gathering, or protest whenever a client is recognized. Though this may assure the therapist that the risk of multiple relationships was prevented, it may be experienced hurtfully by the client as an avoidance or rejection of their presence, particularly when considering the role of rejection sensitivity as a minority stressor for SGM people. The second possibility may be to completely avoid discussing or acknowledging the potential for contact outside of therapy. This is also problematic, as incidental contact may then become a source of awkwardness or confusion for both therapist and client when such contact inevitably occurs. Finally, the therapist may choose to exclude themselves completely from involvement within the broader SGM community. While this would strongly reduce the possibility of encounters outside of therapy, this may be detrimental to the well-being of the SGM therapist.

10.05 Sexual intimacies with current therapy clients/patients

First, let us dispense with the obvious recommendations. Psychologists should not engage sexually with a current client under any circumstances, and it is generally not recommended even after the requisite 2-year period post-therapy given the prior power imbalance and potential for harm to the former client (American Psychological Association, 2017, Standard 10.05). The Ethics Code uses the language "sexual intimacies," however, which may be interpreted broadly. Dating apps popular among both sexual minority men and gender minority people often allow for entering information regarding a variety of sexual preferences, including the user's preferred sexual position. I would recommend that clinically active therapists leave those fields blank. The awareness of a therapist's sexual likes and dislikes, type, or preferred sexual position may increase the likelihood of the sexualization of an ongoing therapeutic relationship.

I have heard a number of anecdotes over the years regarding other ways that therapists manage the risks of such contacts. One that has arisen multiple times is the practice of letting a client know that if you see them on a dating website or app, you will block them and invite them to do the same. While this is a passive action and not visible to other users, the possibility still exists that a client reviews your profile first. For that reason, I still recommend that a therapist consider careful minimization of information included in a profile. Another common report is that a therapist may use a photo that does not clearly show their face, or does not include a photograph of any sort. I would caution against this, as it seems likely to raise the possibility of accidental flirtation before either the client or therapist realizes that they are speaking to one another. I would recommend that if an SGM provider is using a site or app to date or socialize, it would be preferable to be identifiable and sensitive about information made publicly available, rather than anonymous and more likely to have accidental sexual or romantic conversations with clients.

3.05 Multiple relationships and 10.01 informed consent to therapy

Good clinical practice involves a frank discussion of the risks involved as a part of the informed consent process, and management of multiple relationships includes an acknowledgment of areas of overlap where they may occur (American Psychological Association, 2017, Standard 3.05 and 10.01). My former private practice office was located in the middle of the Castro neighborhood, on Castro Street in San Francisco – a location world famous for its association with SGM communities. As a part of the intake process with clients who were members of the community, as well as those who were not but lived nearby, I would introduce the possibility of encountering one another on the street or in restaurants in the neighborhood. Though some SGM clients were initially taken aback, particularly if past SGM therapists had avoided the topic, they were generally grateful to have an open discussion and consider what norms or expectations to have. I would not flee a restaurant, for example. They were welcome to say hello, with the reminder that anyone I was with would be aware of my profession and they would likely be disclosing our relationship. I would also not be the first to approach them or attempt to initiate conversations outside of session.

Though these are only some possible boundaries that a therapist and client may discuss, it is important to consider how they fit within the context of your own life and practice. There may be settings that you feel are too small or intimate, or others such as your place of worship that are irreplaceable. It also may be helpful to seek frequent consultation regarding not only your general practices, but as an adjunct to documenting any extra-therapeutic contacts or conversations with your clients. For example, the risk is two-sided. It is not only possible that a client may interpret your presence as an invitation for a parallel social or romantic relationship, it is also possible that a client may consider your presence an invitation to share a stressor, update the therapist on an ongoing situation, or request support in the moment. These potentialities should be discussed in advance with clients, so that there are shared expectations of what may happen, and clear boundaries around incidental encounters.

2.01 Boundaries of competence and 2.06 personal problems and conflicts

This chapter has barely covered a variety of complex situations that may arise. The final points to consider are the role of boundaries of competence, as well as the guidance of the Ethics Code regarding personal problems and conflicts (American Psychological Association, 2017, Standard 2.01 and 2.06). In a tightly knit lesbian community, for example, does a breakup mean that a sexual minority woman must give up her contact with the local community? If a trans supervisor discovers that the fellow member of a local online forum that they banter with is a current trans supervisee, have they violated the spirit of the Ethics Code or must the student be reassigned? Such situations may not have a simple answer – in the first case, we have circled back to the challenge of an interpretation of the Ethics Code that would isolate a therapist from the community, and in the second, this could lead to denying a trans student the rare opportunity to be supervised by and learn from a trans supervisor, and the growth that would accompany mentorship around unique challenges that arise in the practice of therapy. In both cases, there is little literature for guidance. In these cases, I would recommend consulting with other SGM colleagues in the area who are familiar with local community norms and standards. If this is not possible, there are a number of SGM email lists associated with professional organizations where consultation might be done with someone in a different region of the country. Formal consultation when needed may also be an important additional means of exploring an ethical path forward. Finally, the Ethics Code is clear: if your own difficulties or emotions regarding another person in your capacity as a professional feel too overwhelming to continue the activity, whether with a student, a client, or a colleague, it is your responsibility to withdraw from the environment (American Psychological Association, 2017, Standard 2.06).

Conclusions

It may not be entirely possible within the confines of the SGM community to eliminate all multiple relationships or encounters outside of therapy without the therapist succumbing to isolation and a lack of community support necessary for resilience in their own life. It is also incumbent upon the clinician to be mindful of what multiple relationships might arise. The recent phenomena of dating apps poses certain new challenges, though it is not so unlike other potentially sexualized SGM spaces that decisions cannot be made that would minimize the risk of harm or of inappropriate multiple relationships. Ultimately, it is your responsibility to withdraw from any situation you find yourself in where you feel uncomfortable or unable to discern an ethical path forward.

Key points

- The changing ways that the SGM community engages through apps poses new challenges to navigating multiple relationships.
- SGM therapists should be mindful of the benefits of remaining engaged in the SGM community and attempt to do so in a responsible way.
- If a comfortable resolution is unable to be found, or you experience distress that does not allow you to maintain your professional role, you should remove yourself from that situation.

Recommended reading

American Psychological Association. (2017). Ethical principles of psychologists and code of conduct (2002, amended effective June 1, 2010, and January 1, 2017). https://www.apa.org/ethics/code/.

Fisher, C. B. (2017). *Decoding the ethics code: A practical guide for psychologists* (4th ed.). Sage Publications.

References

American Psychological Association. (2017). Ethical principles of psychologists and code of conduct (2002, amended effective June 1, 2010, and January 1, 2017). https://www.apa.org/ethics/code/.

Berlin, R. (2014). The professional ethics of online dating: Need for guidance. *Journal of the American Academy of Child and Adolescent Psychiatry, 53*(9), 935–937.

Brown, L. S. (1989). Beyond thou shalt not: Thinking about ethics in the lesbian therapy community. *Women & Therapy, 8*(1-2), 13–25.

Campbell, C. D., & Gordon, M. C. (2003). Acknowledging the inevitable: Understanding multiple relationships in rural practice. *Professional Psychology: Research and Practice, 34*(4), 430–434.

Campkin, B., & Marshall, L. (2017). *LGBTQ+ cultural infrastructure in London: Night venues, 2006–present.* UCL Urban Laboratory.

Everett, B., MacFarlane, D. A., Reynolds, V. A., & Anderson, H. D. (2013). Not on our backs: Supporting counsellors in navigating the ethics of multiple relationships within queer, two spirit, and/or trans communities. *Canadian Journal of Counselling and Psychotherapy, 47*(1), 14–28.

Fisher, C. B. (2017). *Decoding the ethics code: A practical guide for psychologists (4th ed.).* Sage Publications.

Gonsiorek, J. C. (1994). *Breach of trust: Sexual exploitation by health care professionals and clergy.* Sage Publications.

Graham, S. R., & Liddle, B. J. (2009). Multiple relationships encountered by lesbian and bisexual psychotherapists: How close is too close? *Professional Psychology: Research and Practice, 40*(1), 15–21.

Guthmann, D., & Sandberg, K. (2002). Dual relationships in the deaf community. In A. Lazarus, & O. Zur (Eds.), *Dual relationships and psychotherapy.* New York, NY: Springer.

Kessler, L. E., & Waehler, C. A. (2005). Addressing multiple relationships between clients and therapists in lesbian, gay, bisexual, and transgender communities. *Professional Psychology: Research and Practice, 36*(1), 66–72.

Lamb, D. H., & Catanzaro, S. J. (1998). Sexual and nonsexual boundary violations involving psychologists, clients, supervisees, and students: Implications for professional practice. *Professional Psychology: Research and Practice, 29*(5), 498.

Mereish, E. H., & Poteat, V. P. (2015). A relational model of sexual minority mental and physical health: The negative effects of shame on relationships, loneliness, and health. *Journal of Counseling Psychology, 62*(3), 425–437.

Morrow, S. L. (2000). First do no harm: Therapist issues in psychotherapy with lesbian, gay, and bisexual clients. In R. M. Perez, K. A. DeBord, & K. J. Bieschke (Eds.), *Handbook of counseling and psychotherapy with lesbian, gay, and bisexual clients* (pp. 137–156). Washington, D.C.: American Psychological Association.

Pflum, S. R., Testa, R. J., Balsam, K. F., Goldblum, P. B., & Bongar, B. (2015). Social support, trans community connectedness, and mental health symptoms among transgender and gender nonconforming adults. *Psychology of Sexual Orientation and Gender Diversity, 2*(3), 281–286.

Robinson, B. A. (2015). "Personal preference" as the new racism: Gay desire and racial cleansing in cyberspace. *Sociology of Race and Ethnicity, 1*(2), 317–330.

Rosenfeld, M. J., & Thomas, R. J. (2012). Searching for a mate: The rise of the Internet as a social intermediary. *American Sociological Review*, *77*(4), 523–547.

Russell, G. M., & Richards, J. A. (2003). Stressor and resilience factors for lesbians, gay men, and bisexuals confronting antigay politics. *American Journal of Community Psychology*, *31*(3-4), 313–328.

Schank, J. A., & Skovholt, T. M. (1997). Dual-relationship dilemmas of rural and small-community psychologists. *Professional Psychology: Research and Practice*, *28*(1), 44–49.

11

FUTURE DIRECTIONS IN SGM THERAPY

Introduction

This book has outlined both a transdiagnostic, process-based approach to psychotherapy with SGM clients as well as a broader consideration of what an affirmative stance by a minority stress-informed clinician might look like in healthcare settings, working with trauma, or in considering an ethical stance that treats SGM clinicians as whole people. A number of questions remain, however, regarding the optimal approach to testing, disseminating, and implementing such an approach. It is also always an interesting experience of emphasizing clinical interventions that serve as a stopgap against the effects of societal bias and violence. The greatest hope and goal would be that such efforts are ultimately unnecessary, and the need for a volume such as this would expire as the world becomes a more inclusive place. There are small rays of hope, such as evidence from Sweden that noted the disappearance of psychological distress disparities between sexual minority people and heterosexuals in response to structural changes in the country in nationwide, population-based surveys (Hatzenbuehler et al., 2018). Though a rare example, the expression "the exception proves the rule" seems apt, as this further supports the assumption in this volume that disparities experienced by SGM people are the result of structural and systemic bias in the external world.

Next steps

While the interventions and techniques described are grounded in a literature developed for general client populations, the use of these techniques has been limited to a handful of pilot studies and unpublished dissertations. Despite this, the use of contextual behavioral approaches with SGM clients has been extended to a variety of SGM client populations and I have been frequently contacted for training and consultation. The resonance or popularity of an approach is not science, however. I am aware of and in some cases a collaborator in a number of trials that explore elements of what is described here, including trials of compassion groups with non-clinical SGM samples and FAP treatment in small trials, that have not yet undergone peer review. I also made the decision early in the preparation of this volume not to include dissertations that have not been translated into peer-reviewed publications, though it is clear from even a cursory review that among future psychologists, contextual approaches that emphasize mindfulness, acceptance, and compassion are incredibly popular. Even if these studies do become disseminated, this still fails to reach the vision of this book of considering how a broader process-based approach that utilizes all of these tools might enhance the well-being of SGM people. Pilots and small sample designs that support these interventions may not guide the evidence-based practitioner in determining the best fit between technique, minority stress target, and client population. Such process-based trials of the broader model are possible, and research on process-based therapies is not the challenge (e.g., Ong et al., 2019). This requires investment by funding agencies, however, and funding for minority health disparities among SGM populations are not current priorities for institutions in which funding for SGM research is often still yoked to HIV prevention science (e.g., Pachankis, 2018).

There are also broader questions about the specifics for each community under the SGM umbrella, which includes cis and trans women and men, non-binary and agender individuals, and sexual minority and gender minority people. One the one hand, the emphasis on the SORC model in this book is intended to highlight the manner in which a contextual behavioral approach should be tailored to each individual. On the other hand, clinical research in this field is still too young to speak with certainty regarding whether targeting specific minority stress components should vary depending on a specific set of identities. While the minority stress model is broadly overlapping across SGM populations, generalization is limited by the recruitment procedures and populations included across studies. Through the development of this model in the United States, nuances are erased that are not global rules, such as the degree to which sexual minority women and men and gender minority people share history. Even as the Mattachine Society and Daughters of Bilitis (the first organizations that grew to a national scale and brought together gay men and lesbians, respectively) saw many of their causes align, with many later groups emphasizing the shared causes of sexual minority women and men, sexual minority advocacy groups in other wealthy nations have not experienced as great a sense of alignment across gender in sexual minority communities (e.g., the United States versus France; Faderman, 2015; Martel, 2000). These differences arise from historical variations in the relation between SGM and women's rights movements, histories of the criminalization of same-sex relationships, and the degree of status of psychiatry in promoting pathologizing models through the 20th century. Similar differences can be found in considering the degree of integration between sexual minority and gender minority communities and sense of shared history. In the United States, the modern LGBTQ+ civil rights movement is often traced to the Stonewall riots that began on June 28, 1969, following the police raid of a bar whose patrons reflected a broad range of SGM people, particularly gender minority people and people of color (Duberman, 2019). That collective history has been reflected in legal battles, with most court cases advancing the rights of both sexual and gender minority people relying on findings of animus and grounded in legislation that prohibits sex discrimination (Diamond & Rosky, 2016). This legal narrative – one in which there is a shared type of SGM history grounded in a society that expresses bias toward those who violate gender-based norms – is deeply grounded in the history of the United States and also may lead a North American science to infer or discover commonality that is not ultimately universal. Other differences include the challenges of healthcare access experienced by gender minority individuals in the United States. The majority of wealthy nations have implemented some form of national healthcare, so it is possible to observe the impact when gender-affirming procedures are nationally available. The first nationwide study of the impact of gender-affirming surgeries, also in Sweden, noted a profound shift in psychological well-being (Bränström & Pachankis, 2020). Psychological wellness disparities remained, albeit at lower levels, and it begs the question of whether trans people in Sweden with different access to medical care may have different needs when seeking competent psychotherapy than a trans individual living in the United States. Finally, though international SGM psychology is in its early stages, and specific commonalities have been noted globally, therapies that meet the needs of SGM people may vary across countries with different histories of rhetoric around gender, sex, and colonization (Horne et al., 2019).

Measuring change

The added challenge exists that there is no single or widely used clinical assessment that would aid a clinician in determining where to begin treatment. While a few attempts have been made, the lack of ongoing clinical data that would determine how sensitive these instruments are to change poses a fundamental barrier, and leaves therapists to resort to traditional outcomes measures that do not yield insight on whether or not the change was specific to changes in components of the minority stress model. One proposed template, the Sexual Minority Stress Scale (SMSS), was drafted by myself and colleagues within the United States but has only been tested and utilized in subsequent research in translation in Poland (e.g., Grabski et al., 2019; Iniewicz et al., 2017). The SMSS has not been used to track clinical change, however, and Iniewicz and colleagues note the challenges of adapting some questions to a national context where living openly and freely disclosing one's sexual orientation remains uncommon (2017). There have also been creative attempts to capture components of the minority stress model that are not often emphasized, such as a newly developed scale that emphasizes the role of shame and pride, though further research is necessary to determine if this measure proves sensitive enough to support clinical tracking of client progress

(Rendina et al., 2019). This is an area of active research, however, and a proposed framework for what would be most meaningful to clinical researchers is beginning to take shape (e.g., Budge et al., 2017). In my own clinical practice, I have attempted to use some promising scales alongside traditional outcomes measures to determine variability over time, though I have found most scales used in minority stress research insensitive to change over time, even in the presence of large shifts in observed behavior.

Training clinicians

Within my own field, psychology, only a small number of programs exist that offer a specialization in SGM health or psychotherapy. Among those, the requirements and quality range drastically. There may be multiple courses that cover SGM psychology and psychotherapy, or a single course. Most include requirements for experience at an SGM-focused training site during an externship year, though I can find no documentation for the programs I have identified that suggest any criteria beyond the population treated and an affirming stance, so no particular type of psychotherapy appears to be emphasized. Many offer mandatory workshops related to SGM psychotherapy, though details are not clear. Some include institutional certifications in LGBTQ mental health, though there is no field consensus in this area in general. The World Professional Association for Transgender Health (WPATH) does offer a path to certification for mental health providers, though the emphasis is on providing gender-affirming care and sufficient knowledge to work with gender minority clients, rather than a particular stance on the approach to therapy within that domain.

This lack of a clear path for training in SGM psychotherapy poses challenges for therapists who wish to grow in this area and are uncertain how to go about this or if the information they receive will lead to improved outcomes in their work with SGM clients. It also may serve to slow the development of intervention science, as there is no common core that the next generation of researchers will have been exposed to. While existing guidelines for practice discussed earlier in this volume may orient clinicians toward the broader issues that they must be aware of, there are still limited resources for the therapist who would like to offer evidence-based interventions that target responses to bias in the lives of SGM people. It is my hope that this volume provides some support for those searching.

Closing thoughts

I hope that this book is not only a helpful resource, but provides inspiration for further research, training, and refinement of how we might best meet the needs of our SGM clients. This is an attempt to integrate the the large body of data supporting minority stress theory with a specific, theory-driven approach to clinical practice. My hope is that our field is beginning to move beyond affirmative practice to embrace more specific therapies that presume an affirmative stance is already present and though necessary, not sufficient. This volume carries my own assumptions and training biases in considering how best to approach minority stress. It has also been shaped by my work as a therapist in private practice, as much outside academia as inside it, and so much by my former students. I hope that it has provided each reader with new tools, or a new way to reflect on old tools, that will enhance your practice and benefit your clients. It is also my hope that it might serve as a foundation for others to build from in the future.

References

Bränström, R., & Pachankis, J. E. (2020). Reduction in mental health treatment utilization among transgender individuals after gender-affirming surgeries: A total population study. *American Journal of Psychiatry*, 177(8), 727–734. https://doi.org/10.1176/appi.ajp.2019.19010080.

Budge, S. L., Israel, T., & Merrill, C. R. S. (2017). Improving the lives of sexual and gender minorities: The promise of psychotherapy research. *Journal of Counseling Psychology*, 64(4), 376–384.

Diamond, L. M., & Rosky, C. J. (2016). Scrutinizing immutability: Research on sexual orientation and US legal advocacy for sexual minorities. *The Journal of Sex Research*, 53(4-5), 363–391.

Duberman, M. B. (2019). *Stonewall: The definitive story of the LGBTQ rights uprising that changed America*. New York, NY: Plume.

Faderman, L. (2015). *The gay revolution: The story of the struggle*. New York, NY: Simon & Schuster.

Grabski, B., Kasparek, K., Müldner-Nieckowski, Ł., & Iniewicz, G. (2019). Sexual quality of life in homosexual and bisexual men: The relative role of minority stress. *The Journal of Sexual Medicine*, 16(6), 860–871.

Hatzenbuehler, M. L., Bränström, R., & Pachankis, J. E. (2018). Societal-level explanations for reductions in sexual orientation mental health disparities: Results from a ten-year, population-based study in Sweden. *Stigma and Health*, *3*(1), 16–26.

Horne, S. G., Maroney, M. R., Nel, J. A., Chaparro, R. A., & Manalastas, E. J. (2019). Emergence of a transnational LGBTI psychology: Commonalities and challenges in advocacy and activism. *American Psychologist*, *74*(8), 967–986.

Iniewicz, G., Sałapa, K., Wrona, M., & Marek, N. (2017). Minority stress among homosexual and bisexual individuals: From theoretical concepts to research tools: The Sexual Minority Stress Scale. *Archives of Psychiatry and Psychotherapy*, *19*(3), 69–80.

Martel, F. (2000). *The pink and the black: Homosexuals in France since 1968*. Stanford, CA: Stanford University Press.

Ong, C. W., Lee, E. B., Krafft, J., Terry, C. L., Barrett, T. S., Levin, M. E., & Twohig, M. P. (2019). A randomized controlled trial of acceptance and commitment therapy for clinical perfectionism. *Journal of Obsessive-Compulsive and Related Disorders*, *22*, 100444.

Pachankis, J. E. (2018). The scientific pursuit of sexual and gender minority mental health treatments: Toward evidence-based affirmative practice. *American Psychologist*, *73*(9), 1207–1219.

Rendina, H. J., López-Matos, J., Wang, K., Pachankis, J. E., & Parsons, J. T. (2019). The role of self-conscious emotions in the sexual health of gay and bisexual men: Psychometric properties and theoretical validation of the sexual shame and pride scale. *The Journal of Sex Research*, *56*(4-5), 620–631.

INDEX

For Product Safety Concerns and Information please contact our EU
representative GPSR@taylorandfrancis.com
Taylor & Francis Verlag GmbH, Kaufingerstraße 24, 80331 München, Germany

www.ingramcontent.com/pod-product-compliance
Lightning Source LLC
Chambersburg PA
CBHW070727220326
41598CB00024BA/3341